THE 100 SIMPLE SECRETS OF
The Best Half of Life

To the residents of Murry Hills

HarperCollins books may be purchased for educational, business, or sales promotional use. For information please write: Special Markets Department, HarperCollins Publishers Inc., 10 East 53rd Street, New York, NY 10022.

HarperCollins Web site: http://www.harpercollins.com

HarperCollins®, ✦®, and HarperSanFrancisco™ are trademarks of Harper-Collins Publishers Inc.

FIRST EDITION

Library of Congress Cataloging-in-Publication Data is available on request.

ISBN 0–06–056473–3 (pbk.)

05 06 07 08 09 RRD(H) 10 9 8 7 6 5 4 3 2

THE 100 SIMPLE SECRETS OF

The Best Half of Life

What Scientists Have Learned
and How You Can Use It

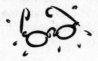

David Niven, Ph.D.

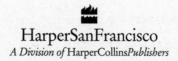

HarperSanFrancisco
A Division of HarperCollins*Publishers*

Contents

Acknowledgments

My thanks to Gideon Weil, Miki Terasawa, Claudia Boutote, Stephen Hanselman, and the many good folks at Harper-SanFrancisco who have worked with me on this book, and to my agent, Sandy Choron. They have helped to make this book a more useful tool for readers, and I offer them my sincere appreciation.

A Note to Readers

Each of the one hundred entries presented here is based on the research conclusions of scientists studying the lives and habits of people in their fifties, sixties, seventies, eighties, and above. Each entry contains a key research conclusion complemented by advice, together with an example that illustrates the conclusion. The research conclusions I present in each entry are based on a meta-analysis of research, which means that each conclusion has been derived from the work of multiple researchers studying the same topic. To enable the reader to find further information on each topic, I have included in each entry a reference to a supporting study. And at the end of the book I have provided a list of sources on happiness over the course of a lifetime.

Introduction

Thinking About Your Future

Nearing retirement after three decades of teaching elementary school students in Ohio, Cathy Martin was thinking a lot about her future. She thought about her plans and priorities for the next phase of her life—where she would live, whether she should work part-time, and where she might travel.

And, to the disappointment of a number of her fifth-grade students no doubt, her thoughts led her to what seemed an interesting and valuable essay assignment. What, she wondered, did her students imagine for their lives when they were in their fifties, sixties, and beyond? Cathy thought the idea of looking many decades ahead in their lives would interest her students and encourage them to think about how their education would contribute to their futures.

In reading the essays, Cathy learned a number of things. "One thing is that almost everybody is convinced we will have some kind of spaceship car that doesn't need wheels and just flies wherever you want to go," Cathy reports.

"The second thing is how much they focused on the action of life. They wrote less about having terrific accomplishments and more about actually doing something terrific. They wrote less about having a stack of money and more about having fun. They wrote less about wanting to have an easy life and more about wanting to have what you might call a full life.

"We adults live our lives with starts and stops," Cathy says. "We start working, we stop working, we start something else. Instead of seeing lots of endings and beginnings, the students saw continuation. They saw a far-off tomorrow as a continuation of today. Nobody wrote about stopping what they wanted to do. Nobody wrote about doing things they didn't think were valuable."

And the students, in writing about the far-off future, were future oriented even about that subject. "They had plans for more—more action, more achievements, more life," she says. "They live in a world where a seventy-seven-year-old man has been an astronaut. They don't see fifty or sixty or seventy as the end of anything at all."

Cathy noticed an absence of negatives in their essays as well: "Nobody focused on disappointments or grudges. And, fortunately, nobody foresaw themselves fifty years later lamenting all the essays their fifth-grade teacher made them write."

Cathy took away a lot from the perspective of her students. "They see themselves as hopeful, excitable, forward looking, and taking action," Cathy says. "They were without dread, without lament, without surrender. And even if they are a bit unrealistic about life, isn't that a wonderful way to approach getting older?"

Cathy resolved to take those lessons to heart, especially as she examined her attitude toward what's next in her own life: "I see my future now more as a step forward instead of a whole new beginning. And I hope I can live up to the expectations of my students for their future lives—except for the part about the space cars."

And in many ways, Cathy's lessons from her students echo some of the most significant research conclusions scientists have drawn regarding happiness over the course of a lifetime. As I conducted the research for *100 Simple Secrets of the Best Half of Life,* reading studies about the habits and practices that contribute to a satisfying life, I found many examples of the great importance of attitudes, perspectives, and a willingness to act. Each entry in *100 Simple Secrets of the Best Half of Life* presents a core research conclusion, an example of the conclusion, and the basic advice experts recommend. I share these findings here for Cathy and for all of you, so that you can use the best scientific information we have to thrive in the best half of your life.

1

Happiness Is Not an Accident

We have strategies for most things in our lives—from work, to games, to how to get home from town two minutes faster. But we leave some of the most important parts of our lives, like our happiness, to chance. Happiness is not like height; you don't just get a certain amount and then have to live with it. Happiness can be improved—if you know what you are doing and what you are not doing, and you care to change.

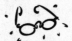

For Patrick, it started with a request from a neighbor. The neighbor had played the part of Santa Claus for several years, creating a tradition of a visit from Santa to all the children in the neighborhood. But one year, Santa had a cold and asked whether Patrick could take over for him that day.

Patrick donned the suit and passed out candy canes and good wishes to all the neighborhood children, calling them each by name and convincing them he was for real. "When I put on the suit, I actually felt like Santa Claus," Patrick says. "It was a truly magical feeling."

When the old Santa saw how much Patrick enjoyed the job, he told Patrick he would be happy to let him take over. Patrick saw the potential for sharing some joy with others and expanded the reach of his duties from his neighborhood to area hospitals. "Sick children would light up when they saw me," Patrick recalls. "I would sit with them, and they would smile from ear to ear. It was such an honor to be able to bring them a good feeling like that."

Over the years the Santa suit wore out and Patrick upgraded to a top-of-the-line model— "the kind they use at the really good malls," he explains.

Patrick has been playing Santa for so long now that he's beginning to see the children of the children he saw as Santa when he first started out. But Patrick has no plans to find a new man for the suit. "Santa never retires," he says.

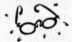

Researchers found that the majority of the subjects they studied were not able to identify anything they had done recently to try to increase their happiness or life satisfaction.

Frijters 2000

2

You Must Approve of Yourself

You can make the best plans in the world for your life. But no action, no accomplishment, no outcome will offer you ultimate fulfillment. You must offer yourself complete, unconditional approval, regardless of whatever takes place in your life.

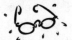

Two of Freddy Johnson's good friends have gone on to become famous and well-paid head coaches in professional and college basketball. Freddy coaches boys' high school basketball on a far smaller stage, for a far smaller paycheck.

Far from being jealous of his friends or disappointed in himself, Freddy celebrates their successes and his own. He saves newspaper clippings about his old friends and keeps them in his office for the players he coaches and his visitors to see.

And Freddy never doubts the value of having spent almost three decades teaching and coaching the game. "It's amazing where some of the guys I know are now," he says. "But I'm happy where I am, too. I wouldn't trade it for the world." Freddy has coached teams that have won more than six hundred games and a half dozen state titles.

Freddy's fellow high school coaches admire his willingness to keeping learning. "He never stops soaking up basketball knowledge," says one colleague. "There's always a game to watch somewhere, another insight to be gained." But most of all, his peers admire his willingness to surround himself with good people. As the colleague puts it, "Head coaches always want to be the dominant force on their team. No one else should know as much as they do. No one else should question decisions that are made. But Freddy seeks to be around the best assistants in the game because he has the self-confidence to surround himself with talented people and to take their success as something he, too, can be proud of."

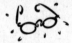

Those who considered themselves a success were 25 percent less likely to feel anxious about their lives, 14 percent less likely to be selfish, and 45 percent more likely to say they enjoyed their lives.

Chamberlain and Haaga 2001

3

Keep Going

It's hard to get much done one little step at a time. But it's impossible to get anything significant accomplished without going one little step at a time. The capacity to continue, to move forward despite obstacles, becomes even more important as we age. Even though there may not be projects at work or deadlines to face, the need to fight through obstacles and move toward your desired outcome serves every part of your life.

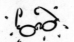

Just out of medical school, Dr. Robert Lopatin was working hundred-hour weeks as a first-year medical resident. Unlike other residents, who often drew skeptical looks from patients wondering if the residents were really old enough to be doctors, Robert seemed to inspire a calm confidence. In fact, not a single patient questioned whether he was old enough be a doctor.

It could have had something to do with the fact that he was fifty-five years old.

As a boy, Robert had imagined himself as a doctor. But when he was in school his father asked him to join him in a new clothing business he was starting. And for almost three decades, Robert dedicated himself to the business.

But when his father sold the business to a competitor, the newly unemployed Robert knew exactly what he wanted to do with his time: go back to school. After trying several areas of study, he realized that his desire to be a doctor was still as strong as it had been when he was a boy.

At age fifty-one Robert began studying at the Albert Einstein College of Medicine in New York City. He was older than most of his professors. He was even older than the school itself. But he felt completely at ease. "It took a lot of imagination to do it, but once I undertook it, it just felt so right," he says. "I felt I was home again."

Dr. Lopatin now practices in New York. And he encourages others to keep going, even if they didn't quite get where they were heading when they were younger: "When you're older, once you do make a commitment to something, there's more purposefulness and there's more joy."

People in their sixties and beyond who had a long-term plan to accomplish something were 31 percent more likely to report that they enjoyed their lives.

Wallace, Bisconti, and Bergeman 2001

4

Try Something New

We are often leery of new things—whether they're as important as a new job or a new direction in life, or as trivial as a new product in the supermarket—because we are comfortable with the old and familiar. Give yourself a chance to try new things. They won't always be what you want, but it's unlikely they won't ever be what you want.

Lisa knows it's not the typical path. "Most people, when they graduate from high school, don't ever want to come back," she says. Instead, the sixty-something mother and grandmother decided to return to high school, as a substitute teacher, four decades after she graduated. Substitute teaching was just the thing to give her some variety in her life while still leaving her with free time.

Lisa says she likes the idea that every day is a little different and holds something new. "And I feel needed," she adds. "I fill a void. It's my contribution to the world."

Interacting with different generations also is energizing for her: "I really like young people. They give me a fresh outlook. I like to do anything the students do. In math, which is not my strongest subject, I have great respect for their knowledge. And I learn new things in the process. It's exercise for my brain, and it's a joy.

"I think I'm a student at heart. I have an insatiable quest for knowledge, reviewing what I studied years ago and learning new material and then teaching it. It's a great way to learn.

"Sometimes when I get home from school my friends ask, 'When are you going to stop that foolishness?' But it's not foolishness. It's fun."

Those over fifty who showed a high degree of resistance to change were 26 percent less likely to feel optimistic about their futures.

Caughlin and Golish 2002

5

You Still Are Who You Were

Pick up an article about advertising and demographics, and you will learn that to some industries, the only people who matter are no older than forty, or thirty, or even twenty-five. There is no shortage of cultural bellwethers suggesting that we are most interesting and useful when we are young. It's almost as if we come with an expiration date for cultural relevance. As arbitrary as these notions are, we can arm ourselves with the best defense possible against feeling out-of-date. In truth, we are every age we've ever been. We have all the experiences of a forty-year-old, a thirty-year-old, a twenty-five-year-old within us. Let yourself think about all that you've known and done, and, far from feeling out-of-date, you will feel even better about who you are today.

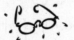

She had spent her career in education, teaching and eventually serving as a principal. In her spare time she had served countless community groups, from the Boy Scouts to Habitat for Humanity. But Rebecca Adams felt she could do more for her community.

She'd never done anything like it before, but at the age of fifty-seven, Rebecca decided she wanted to run for city council in her hometown of Chesapeake, Virginia.

Against the advice of local political experts, she entered the field of fifteen candidates, all seeking one seat. "Nobody out and out said, 'You're too old,'" she recalls, "but people said things like 'Is this really what you want to do with your time and energy at this point?' And I said yes.

"People think you should slow down when you're staring sixty in the face. But you don't have to slow down if you don't spend your time thinking about turning sixty. We all have the same 10,080 minutes in a week," Rebecca says. "We can spend them worrying about getting old, or we can do something more productive with them."

Though she very much wanted to win the election and serve her city, her expectations were modest. "I honestly thought I would finish seventh or eighth," Rebecca says.

She ran her campaign with no experience and little money but with lots of hard work. And she won. Now, with a seat on the city council, she has her mind firmly focused in one direction. "We've got to decide what we want to look like in the future," Rebecca says, referring both to her hometown and to its people.

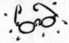

Those who strongly identified with their current age became 2 percent less satisfied with their lives with every passing year, while those who infrequently thought in terms of their age showed no such negative trend.

Reis-Bergan et al. 2000

6

Happy Looks for Happy

If you are convinced that things are bad, you will notice many unpleasant things and unpleasant people. If you are convinced that things are good, you will notice many pleasant things and pleasant people. Understand that every one of us selectively perceives the world around us. We see far too many things every time we step outside the door to focus on all of them. You can get all the supporting evidence you want, regardless of whether you start today determined to think the worst of the world or determined to think the best.

The breeze comes in softly as the sun sets. Chris looks out, and as far as the eye can see stretches the calm blue ocean. In the distance, ships passing miles out from the coast come into view. Chris works at a Florida lighthouse. He knows every inch of the place, exactly how everything works.

Chris came to the lighthouse after serving for more than two decades as a New York City firefighter.

He wasn't on duty on September 11, 2001, but he raced into lower Manhattan to try to serve. Reaching the Twin Towers after they had collapsed, he found a devastated area that looked like a war zone. The ash and smoke were overwhelming.

It was spooky, Chris says, because there were fire trucks everywhere, but no firemen. Only later did he realize the nature of the devastation suffered by the fire department, including the loss of one of his closest friends.

He mourned, feeling survivor's guilt and slipping deeper into gloom. Everywhere in the city, even in his home, were reminders of that day. He left the department—not to forget, but to find another way.

Chris and his family decided that a move to Florida was the right thing. Now he takes solace in adjusting to the rhythms of a new work routine, meeting new neighbors, and doing some of the things you can do in Florida that you just can't farther north, like going kayaking in January.

Researchers who studied people's level of interest in and attention to strangers found that people who were sad spent 35 percent more time focusing on strangers who looked unhappy than on strangers who looked happy.

Gotlib et al. 2004

7

The Mirror Will Be Kinder

How we feel about our bodies has a lot to do with how we feel about ourselves. Whether we see ourselves as strong and capable, even whether we see ourselves as kind and competent, is related to our personal body image. The good news is that, contrary to the widespread fear that we will be less and less pleased with our bodies as we get older, we actually become more positive about them. We begin to see character where we once saw only flaws. We begin to see strength where we once saw only weakness. We begin to see ourselves where we once saw only the image of what we thought we should look like.

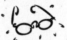

In 1999, a women's group in Rylstone, England, decided not to continue featuring pictures of well-kept landscaped grounds on its annual fund-raising calendar. Instead, members of the women's group, ranging in age from forty-five to sixty-six, posed in the buff for the calendar.

Sales of the calendar, which in previous years the group hoped would bring in two thousand dollars, that year amounted to more than one million dollars for leukemia charities.

Interestingly, the calendar sold well with both men and women. Women thought it was a tasteful and fun celebration of women's bodies. And men responded to the depiction of what they consider to be real women. As one man said, "How wonderful to see real women instead of stick insects with pouty lips and pipe cleaners for legs."

The calendar and its participants later inspired the film *Calendar Girls.*

As sociologist Ann Morgan argues, "Whether posing nude is a giant step forward is no doubt a whole other debate. But in claiming and proclaiming their bodies for themselves—and, by extension, for others—these women have made a very positive gesture. The notion of a beautiful body image must be understood not for the exclusivity of beauty, but for its variety."

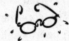

People become about 1 percent more likely to hold a positive image of their bodies with each year of age after forty.

Reboussin et al. 2000

8

Fun Is Not Over

Fun is for young people. They have the time, they have the opportunity, they have the ability. Those may be common assumptions, but none are true. Though the source of fun and happiness may change over the course of our lives, our ability to have fun and our interest in doing so are in no way reduced as we age.

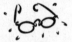

Seventy-four-year-old Jack McKeon has spent nearly all of his adult life involved in major-league baseball. He has run teams from the dugout and from the front office.

In 2003, he was out of baseball. "I wasn't retired," he says, "just in between jobs."

Then, two months into the baseball season, the Florida Marlins called. They needed a new manager who could turn the team's fortunes around. Immediately.

With no hesitation, Jack took the job, becoming the third-oldest manager in baseball history.

He found himself surrounded by ballplayers younger than his grandchildren. But he had no fear that he could no longer relate to young players. In fact, "being around these guys has made me a young kid again," Jack says. "I feel so young, I quit using my senior-citizen discount at restaurants."

Jack still has a serious competitiveness and work ethic that motivate him to show up at the stadium ten hours before a game. And he expects his players to share that drive. But he never lets himself or his players forget that "baseball should be fun." He says, "If you are happy and relaxed, you thrive. If you are a tense perfectionist, this game will break you down."

Jack's team hardly broke down: he led the Marlins to a World Series victory in 2003.

Studies have shown that each additional enjoyable activity that people over fifty engage in per month increases their likelihood of life satisfaction by 2 percent.

Cameron 1972

9

See the Beauty Around You

It could be a flower. It could be a work of art. It could be the great-est pass you've ever seen a quarterback throw. Whatever it is you appreciate, take time to truly see the things that inspire you. Take time to fit them into your life every day. There is beauty in the world around you, however you define it, and wonder, awe, and inspiration are the elixirs of life.

David gave his wife roses on their anniversary. But he saw them from a whole different vantage point than most people.

Looking at the flowers in a vase, the amateur photographer wondered what kind of picture he might be able to create if he took an extreme close-up of a single perfect rose petal. He positioned his camera only inches away from the flowers and created a photo in which one petal fills the entire frame.

When he saw the developed photo, he was excited: "The close-up has the effect of distorting what you are looking at. If you didn't know it was a rose petal, you wouldn't immediately recognize what it was. When it becomes abstract like that, I think, it reveals a different kind of beauty than what you had with the entire flower."

Although he wasn't sure others would appreciate the photo, he submitted it to an art show, and it was accepted. "I thought, 'They can't possibly be interested in it,'" David recalls, "but they saw something in it."

David dedicates most of his photographic efforts to nature scenes. Nature photography, he thinks, is a more creative process, one that requires him to really stop, soak in his environment, and hone in on the beauty in it.

"And," he adds, "unlike people, seldom do trees complain that you didn't get them from a flattering angle."

Those who said they regularly took notice of something beautiful were 12 percent more likely to say they were satisfied with their lives.

Isaacowitz, Vaillant, and Seligman 2003

10

Never Retire from Life

Regardless of when you retire, your first priority in retirement must be to activate yourself. Retirement can be anything from the greatest celebration of life to a dreary bore, depending on the person. Those who allow themselves to wallow in retirement tend to lose focus, finding the hours impossible to fill. Those who are invigorated by retirement embrace the possibilities newly available to them, finding themselves doing as much as they did while working, or even more. Retirement is freedom, but freedom is useful only if you do something with it.

Jane Pauley was in front of the cameras on the *Today* show and *Dateline* for more than twenty-five years. Then she retired from television.

Despite the appearance that she was escaping television's pressures, she never intended to go very far. "When I left *Dateline*, I did not know what I was going to do. I knew I was going to do something, and I knew it was time to do something different. I did not want to retire from life," Jane says.

She sought work that reflected her passions and interests: "What I've learned is if I'm going to work, to be its best, it had better be work I choose."

Jane spent months working on a memoir of her life in television that had been lying around unfinished in her study. And she began planning a new talk show. She describes the more than a year she spent planning the show before it went on the air as being like a "fifteen-month pregnancy."

Jane's talk show is a step away from the news programming she spent her career in, and for the first time, she is working in front of a studio audience. Jane says the new format is both a great challenge and a source of inspiration: "I don't think I understood how important working with an audience would be to me. I love it. I take chances because I know the people in the audience want to see something different and real. I chose to do this show because, even with the pressures, it fits who I am, what I do best, and what I want to do at this point in my life. I've discovered I'm more of a performer than I realized I was."

Recent retirees were 15 percent more likely to be happy than those of a similar age who continued working full-time, but within six months retirees' happiness fell behind that of those of a similar age who were working if the retirees did not have an active lifestyle.

Wells and Kendig 1999

11

Have Time for Thoughts

We have the capacity to have deep, moving, insightful thoughts about our lives and the world around us. But our daily habits, routines, and responsibilities often soak up our available time and attention. Give yourself the opportunity to think, to question, and to ponder, and you will enjoy not only the fruits of an occasional good idea but the joy of thought itself.

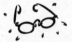

At seventy-eight, Harry took his thirty-two-foot sailboat out for a trip . . . around the world. At eighty-eight, he thought it was time to circle the globe again. "I like being alone at sea," he says. "I like the challenge of ocean crossing. I'm always delighted to be back among people, but after a while, I wish I was back at sea again.

"The way to stay young is to stay active physically and mentally. If you're sailing the seas, you have to be constantly engaged in the process."

But in calm waters Harry can afford to take some time to read the history, poetry, and mystery books he brings with him on board, listen to whatever news reports he can pick up on the radio, and think. "There's plenty of time for reflecting on things when you are out there," he says.

Harry's trips are not just about being at sea. When he reaches a port, he likes to explore the area. A small village in Japan even threw a celebration for him, sending area schoolchildren to greet Harry upon his arrival and to listen to him speak of his adventures.

A retired chemist, Harry focused on creating long-range research plans for his company while he was working. And he's still making long-range plans for himself. But he thinks this will be his last trip around the world. "After all," he says, "the boat's getting pretty old."

People who said they were very busy or stressed were 17 percent less likely to say they felt that they adequately thought through the decisions they made.

Bippus and Rollin 2003

12

Turn Off the Bad News

It's not news when a plane lands safely or a bank isn't robbed. The nature of news is to focus on what's different and what's unexpected. Unfortunately, all too often that results in a newscast made up of a list of bad things that have happened to people. Be mindful that the television news is only a slice of the world—usually not the most pleasant slice—and give yourself ample opportunity to see life from a different perspective.

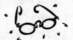

Studying how people spent their time was something Bob Stanley did as part of his job as a psychology professor.

He was particularly interested in the effects of people's workdays on how they related to others and to their families. "It was a natural extension of some of the same issues I was facing in my life," he says. "And I applied what I observed about myself and my friends to help create my research plan."

Once he retired, Bob was again struck by an observation from his own life: "I like to watch the news. When I was working, I used to watch once a day. But now that I have more free time, I might watch some news in the morning, then again at lunchtime, then at night. And I began to think about how many sad and hopeless things were happening in front of me every night: wars, famines, natural disasters. And I thought about the effect watching all that sadness was having on me."

Bob quietly observed some of his friends and found that their news-viewing habits were often similar to his. Without worrying about all the details that would go into a full-scale research project, he decided to try a little experiment.

For several days, he participated in conversations with his friends on whatever topic might come up. Bob quietly noted how many times he and his friends led the conversation to negative topics, whether personal or news related. Later, he asked each of his friends to skip watching any television news for three days. He told them it was part of a study of current-events knowledge. After the three days, Bob again spoke to his friends and noted how many negative topics came up.

"It turns out my friends spent half as much time talking about negative topics when they hadn't seen television news for a few days," Bob reports. When he came clean about his experiment with his friends, they wanted to know if it was all right for them to continue reading the newspaper. Bob said, "I think so. I could run some more tests if you'd like."

People who consumed high levels of television news were twice as likely to have negative feelings about the direction the world is taking.

Pinkleton and Austin 2002

13

Express Yourself in What You Do

Do something today that reflects who you are, what you are capable of, and what you care about. Whether at work or at home, for pay or for free, do something that reflects you. We need to see evidence of our abilities; we need to see evidence of our relevance. Once you give yourself proof of what you can do, you will not doubt your ability to do anything.

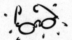

Larry Brody wrote for numerous televisions shows, including *Baretta, Barnaby Jones, Diagnosis Murder, Hawaii Five-O, The Six Million Dollar Man,* and *Walker, Texas Ranger.*

But one of the greatest joys of his career in television was working with other writers, particularly those just starting out. "There is so much untapped talent out there," he says. "I loved to help new colleagues grow into the role of being a writer."

Larry decided he wanted to go into semiretirement to get away from the stress of Hollywood life. A friend had recommended he consider Arkansas. And though he'd never been there, he visited and was soon convinced it was the right place for him.

Still, he wanted to continue to help young writers. From his Arkansas ranch he has organized a variety of opportunities for young writers to have their work critiqued, including contests for scripts and short films. Larry offers feedback based on his understanding of the fundamentals of writing: "If you've got the pacing and the rhythm, you've got half of it. If you have that, and something you want to share, you're just about there."

The point of Larry's efforts is to nurture talent. "It's all about dreams—about making dreams come true," he says. In fact, at this point he gets more satisfaction from contributing to other writers than he does from writing itself. "I'd rather teach other people to put it together than do anything else in the business," he says.

People who felt they had an outlet for self-expression were 19 percent more likely to feel confident about themselves and 18 percent more likely to feel satisfied with their lives.

Christiansen 2000

14

You Are Not Old

Everybody likes to disparage old things. Nobody wants old news, old bread, or old anything. But wait. People love antique tables. People love vintage cars. Old tables and old cars are things bound for the dump, but change your perspective and you have something more valuable and cherished than even something new. You are not old; you are not yesterday's news or day-old bread. See the value in who you are and what you are.

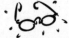

"I became a bachelor again after age fifty-five. Some people would think, 'Well, that's about that.' Ha! The fun's just starting," says Tom.

Tom started dating again, aided by an Internet personals service. "You ask for a certain age, location, personality—what have you. And you get back one hundred women in your area," Tom reports. "That's a lot of choice and a lot of possibility."

Tom has many friends who have used the personals services, and it hasn't always worked out: "One poor fellow found a woman and set up a date over email. Showed up to meet the woman for coffee and found he had accidentally asked his ex-wife out on a date."

And Tom says most people "lie about their age, by three to five years. So I knock off five years just to get even."

Still, Tom says he has met some wonderful people and been amazed at the way deep, personal relationships can be built online. "You have all these conversations over email. It's not just that you both 'like skiing' and you both 'like tofu,'" he says. "It goes much deeper than that."

More than anything, he sees the people online as "so alive—alive with possibility. There aren't any listings from people calling themselves old and defeated."

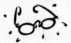

People over age fifty who did not think of themselves as old were 39 percent more likely to be happy.

Hurd 1999

15

Money Can't Buy Happiness

Name the happiest day of your life. For almost everyone, that day had nothing to do with money. Yet we spend much of our work time and free time directed toward money: making more, getting more, keeping more, and spending more. Money is necessary for the basics of life, to be sure, but increasing sums of money do not increase our enjoyment of life—just our desire for more money.

Tennessee resident Kim Hunt knows what it's like to become a millionaire in an instant. A contestant on the game show *Who Wants to Be a Millionaire,* Kim answered fourteen questions correctly and then answered the million-dollar question.

The veteran math teacher in his forties went from living on a very modest salary to having a pile of money at his disposal. Kim's first priority was to help his parents. They had provided so much for him, helping him through college, and they were now struggling with medical bills. "I was always the professional student. Always the one without money," Kim recalls. "So it was nice to be able to do something for them."

Then he purchased some things he really wanted: a new computer and a new car.

But he soon realized that, with few exceptions, he was "pretty much living my old lifestyle. The money changes less than you might think. Some people ask me for money when they never did before. But I get up in the morning and I'm still the same person."

One thing that has changed, ironically, is that Kim spends more time worrying about money: "I didn't have any before, and I didn't think much about it. Now I'm trying hard not to do something really stupid and lose all the money. I've got it socked away in stocks and mutual funds—which, sadly, have actually lost some value since I bought them."

People's ratings of their own happiness do not increase as their income rises, because their appetite for products increases along with their income.

Easterlin 2001

16

The Only Requirement Is Embracing the Lack of Requirements

Will early retirement meet your needs? Will working long past when you could retire make you happy? The answer is that either path is available and can make people happy. Do not try to fit yourself into a pattern or timetable. Embrace the value of the choices available to you.

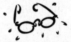

Terry remembers well the feeling of *What's next?* as his career as a career counselor approached its end. He says, "There are a lot of expectations on you when you're younger, but you reach a certain age and you find there are no expectations at all. Then, if you are not careful, it's as if you sit around waiting for an invitation to do something."

Terry says that the way we live our lives makes contemplating transitions and new directions all the more difficult: "We're always in a hurry, running through life. Then we step out of that life and find we're not ready for what's next."

Events and milestones are often used as the starting point for a new assessment of oneself, he says, but there is no need to wait: "Think about it right now. You don't need to wait until your last child moves out the door, until you retire, until you sell the house and move to a condo in Florida. Think about what you want to do with your life right this very minute."

Thinking about what's next is often a basic matter of connections. "To what, to whom do you feel connected? What is it that inspires you, that brings you joy?" Terry asks. "When you become aware of that, and that sense of connection becomes part of you, your next step will be clear."

Terry argues that, although it can be unsettling, the process of defining our direction later in life makes us "more of who we really are. We're more complete. And that makes our time, whether structured or unstructured, more fulfilling."

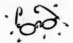

In studies of people in their fifties and older, there was no consistent difference in life satisfaction between those who worked full-time, those who worked part-time, and those who did not work at all.

Fouquereau, Fernandez, and Mullet 2001

17

Keep Your Fears in Line

A large part of our lives is spent imagining the worst that can happen and its consequences. Step back from your fears and worries, and realize that one of the biggest hurdles to overcome is not what you are afraid of but the very fact that you are afraid.

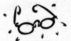

"I guess I'm really the ultimate example of worrying yourself sick," says Marty.

Concerned about a persistent cough for which doctors could offer no relief or explanation, Marty sought second, third, and fourth opinions. On the day he had an appointment to get yet another opinion, a snowstorm blanketed his town. Rather than reschedule, Marty insisted on clearing off his driveway so he could head out to keep his appointment.

The combination of snow and ice made for tough going, and in an effort to gain some traction Marty fell and landed on his arm. "Well, I was going to the doctor, there was no doubt about that," he recalls. "Only then I thought it might be an orthopedist instead."

Marty had broken his arm. After a trip to the hospital, he returned in a cast.

With other things on his mind now, Marty canceled the appointment he was trying to get to in the first place. After a few weeks of rest, he found that his cough was gone but his arm very much still broken.

Marty has extracted two lessons from his experience. First: when it snows, stay inside. Second: worrying is more trouble than it's worth. "I think of it as kind of like that old saying 'Laugh and the whole world laughs with you. Cry, and I'll give you something to cry about,'" he adds.

Relative to the opinions of their own doctors, most people were four times more likely to think of themselves as likely to suffer a debilitating illness in the near future.

Sarkisian et al. 2001

18

Sign Up for Everything

High school kids across the land are busy signing up for the school paper, the debate club, and the basketball team. You may think that now that you're older, those days are gone. The truth is that throwing yourself into as many activities as you can—be they social, athletic, civic, or whatever else interests you—is even more valuable for you now than it was in high school. Activities exercise the brain, forge strong social ties, and improve the disposition.

Manny doesn't understand the image many people have of retirement. "I'm not grumpy or slow, and I don't even own a rocking chair, much less spend all day in it," says the eighty-five-year-old.

Manny has retired from two careers, but he keeps his days full with training for the Senior Olympics, working part-time, and entering his artwork in competitions. In fact, Manny has had fun with so many activities that the only thing that limits him is time: "I had to quit softball a few years ago because it conflicted with my tennis."

Manny not only plays tennis but has also served as a ball "boy" at the U.S. Open. "You know those kids you see scurrying after the ball when it hits the net? That's me," he explains. The only difference is that Manny became the oldest ball boy ever to serve at the tournament. Manny doesn't want attention for his age, though. "That's all overrated," he says. "I think age is a state of mind."

Nevertheless, he realizes that people half his age may spend their time doing far less than half of what he does in a day. But Manny says the value of staying busy is clear regardless of age: "If you sit around, you have time to think about your problems."

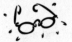

Research on people in their fifties and older found that each group activity that they engaged in per week increased the likelihood of life satisfaction by 3 percent.

McGuinn and Mosher-Ashley 2000

19

Be Decisive

We can actually suffer from having too many alternatives when we make a decision. Our lives are loaded with alternatives. We can follow almost an infinite number of directions. How can we be sure we pick the best one? We can't be. The task is to make the best decision we can and then stop questioning it.

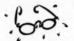

Karen was offered the opportunity to participate in an early retirement program. She saw the pros and the cons all too well: "I think I would enjoy a sort of semi-retirement, or a temporary retirement. But this is all or nothing. Stay, and keep doing my full-time job, or go, and leave this job completely behind."

Each day for a month she tossed the idea around. "I was like a car spinning its wheels," she recalls. "There was an awful lot of effort, and absolutely no progress."

Karen was stymied by what is theoretically the great gift of being her age. "There aren't any rules," she says. "Up to this point, there have been rules—things you are supposed to do. Now, here, I find myself with no rules whatsoever. What are you supposed to do? Nobody has the faintest idea."

Karen eventually said no to early retirement, reasoning that if she couldn't decide whether to retire in the first place, she would have an even harder time deciding what to do with that retirement. "I felt instantly better when I had made a decision. It was like being a little kid in school—staring at a multiple-choice question and debating whether to change your answer. Now that I've finally turned in my paper, I don't really worry so much about my score."

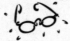

Second-guessing your decisions on a regular basis reduces by 26 percent the likelihood of your believing in your own capabilities.

Bargdill 2000

20

Believe You Can

We love tests and contests. We want to know who is better, in everything from spelling to sprinting. We embrace the certainty that everything can be measured and that the results will tell us who can do what. Unfortunately, there are no tests for the most important things in life. Your ability to thrive as you age, as you retire, as you start seeking a new path in life cannot be predicted by your grades in school or your evaluations on the job. You simply have to believe in yourself—believe in the abilities, the vision, the passion, the core that brought you this far. There is no test. And that is unnerving—but it is also empowering.

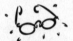

Jeanne knows something about living in a land of tests without really knowing where you rank. Jeanne has spent her working life teaching drama to high school students.

"Unlike the math teacher, who not only can tell you whether you are doing well but can give you an exact percentage for everything you do, all I can do is tell my students to embrace a process," Jeanne says. After all, even the greatest performance "is not something tangible; it's the magic that happens between a performer and an audience."

The same is true for her teaching. "I have an enthusiasm for giving to my students in the classroom and in rehearsals," she says, "but if you said, 'Show it to me on a piece of paper,' I couldn't."

Though she wanted to become an actress, Jeanne embraced the rewards of teaching: "It wasn't the glamour and the spectacle that I had set out for, but it had its own kind of excitement: giving students an opportunity, giving them a challenge, and watching their confidence grow."

Despite the lack of tests and paperwork, Jeanne won an award as teacher of the year. The award cited her for "bringing students into a theater experience in which they find they are capable in ways they never before imagined."

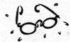

Among those soon to retire or newly retired, a belief in personal capability increased feelings of optimism for the future by 37 percent and increased feelings of happiness by 52 percent.

Efklides, Kalaitzidou, and Chankin 2003

21

See the Real Pay in Work

Asked to define the rewards of work, people first think of money. But for most of us, the value of work is not merely a paycheck but a host of personal and social rewards that make us feel we've accomplished something and are part of a team. When evaluating your career plans, don't lose sight of what it really is that you get from a job.

Psychologist Sandy Lyons has studied retirees to get a better understanding of how people truly feel about their work.

"You can ask people about their jobs, but they are so caught up in the daily reality of work that they can hardly see how they really feel. It's like asking someone how they feel about air. It's all around them, but they've never given it the first thought," she says.

That's why Dr. Lyons looks at how people respond to the absence of a job. "What you tend to see in retirees," she says, "is a frustration about not knowing how they are of value anymore and, even more often, a sense of isolation.

"We think of work as providing for our most basic needs regarding an income, an ability to provide for our family. But at the same time, work provides for even more basic needs in making us feel connected to something, to others."

Dr. Lyons says the retirees who walk away from work cold turkey tend to suffer the most. "Leaving a job as if you are just flipping off a switch can be very painful," she says, "because it dramatically takes away so much of who you are." Dr. Lyons says that people who instead transition out of work by gradually cutting their hours, maintaining contact with some co-workers, and maintaining some connection to their previous work have an easier time building a new life experience for themselves.

All this, Dr. Lyons says, is valuable not just for retirement planning but for career planning: "We should all learn from retirees that we should be thinking in terms of having work meet our basic needs."

Studies of people over the age of fifty-five who work show that 46 percent find their interactions with their co-workers the most rewarding aspect of the job—twice as many as say that their salary is the most rewarding part of the job.

Kaye, Alexander, and Kauffman 1999

22

Know Your Health

The less we know about something, the more we are subject to its vagaries. In ancient times, the Incas and the Aztecs feared comets because they did not understand their movements. Etruscans feared the weather because its patterns of change were so ill understood. Knowing more about your health, both when something ails you and when you feel fine, not only will help you choose a healthy lifestyle but will reduce your fears of a health-related impediment to the quality of your life.

For Barbara Pariente, being nominated as a justice of the Florida Supreme Court represented an unbelievable triumph, the culmination of a law career during which she came across few women colleagues. The court hears some of the most controversial cases in the nation, and she holds one of its seven seats.

As a lawyer and as a judge, she never shied away from the challenge of taking on complex cases and understanding countless details.

When she found out she had breast cancer, she reacted in the same way. "I wanted to learn everything I could," she says. "The first thing I learned was that you may be fearful, but you will be able to come through it and not only survive but thrive."

After her initial diagnosis, Barbara threw herself into a mini-medical school curriculum. When tests to determine if the cancer had spread were inconclusive, it was Barbara who guided her doctors toward further tests, which revealed that the cancer was in the initial stages of spreading.

Even with a complete diagnosis, Barbara received varied recommendations on treatment from her team of more than a dozen doctors. She took it upon herself to sift through their advice and arrive at the best treatment. She chose a very aggressive response to the cancer.

For Barbara, getting all the information she could was empowering. "You can say either 'I'm going to give in to this disease' or 'I'm going to confront it and beat it,'" she says. And now, with her cancer in remission, she adds, "I can't say I'm glad I had cancer. But I'm not sad I had cancer. I am healthy. I am surviving. I am thriving."

People who took an active interest not only in their illnesses but in their overall health were 15 percent more likely to feel that any health problems they had were not reducing their life satisfaction.

Othaganont, Sinthuvorakan, and Jensupakarn 2002

23

See a New Way

When the easy answers have been tried and the problem remains, the time is ripe for your creative powers. Be willing to look at things in a new way, think about them with a fresh perspective, and tap the hidden ideas within yourself.

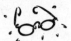

Gerry was an executive with a major financial company. Every day was stressful and long, and featured a brutal commute. "At some point you have to ask yourself why are you doing this," Gerry says.

Offered the opportunity to head his hometown's YMCA, Gerry jumped at the chance—despite a dramatic cut in pay.

His commute is now three minutes long, and his days are stress free. But more important than those things, Gerry says, is that the career switch has given him the chance to make a difference in his community; "Every day I'm thinking about how to serve people through this organization. A good decision doesn't shift the marginal return rate on some unseen transaction. A good decision serves a person who lives right down the street.

"In the corporate world, I saw it as important for me to do as well as I could do financially," Gerry says. "But now I realize it's important for me to be closer to home, to do something that really resonates with me today in terms of my values.

"I realize this doesn't match the corporate world in pay, but neither can the corporate world feed my spirit as much as this does."

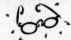

Among those experiencing low life satisfaction, a willingness to think creatively about their problems was associated with an 11 percent shorter duration of negative feelings.

Zhou and George 2001

24

Avoid Generational Competition

Generations see things differently because of changes in the culture, because of changes in events, and sometimes just because they can. Accepting different generational perspectives as a reality of life, rather than feeling a sense of rivalry against those with different views, allows us to continue functioning in an evolving world even as we continue to value our own perspectives.

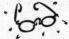

"I have experience. I have opinions. And I probably push too far," Lynn says in explaining why she's taking a class in grandparenting at her local community center.

Lynn told her daughter one too many times about the proper way to dress a child or the level of table manners expected of a child. Tensions rose, and her family could seldom enjoy each other's company. "Each time, I thought I knew best." Lynn recalls. "I was trying to help her head off mistakes. Because what's the point of making a mistake if you don't have to?"

But the lessons she's learning in grandparenting class are offering Lynn a new perspective. "They say we grandparents can push for too much control," Lynn reports. According to the class, she says, "grandparents have to leave their egos at the door and not try to impose their parental perspective on their adult offspring. We've always thought we're the most important generation ever and everything revolves around us and we've figured everything out. And we need to know that not everyone is going to see eye-to-eye with us. And that's not their fault."

Because of the class, Lynn will never again say, "I know what to do. I raised you," she avows. "I guess it's kind of demeaning and demanding: 'Do everything my way because I've done this before.' But it's tough. I'm still having to edit myself."

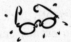

Nine in ten parents said there were significant differences in their approach to parenting compared with that of their parents, and the majority said these differing approaches were a source of intergenerational tension.

Morman and Floyd 2002

25

Respond to Stress

Stress is an accumulation of events and circumstances that represent more than we can handle. Stress eats away at our body's ability to function both mentally and physically. The best response to stress is not to push yourself and wait for it to go away, but rather to try to reduce stress, both by avoiding the circumstances that are causing it and by creating healthier outlets for the pressures in your life.

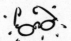

Ruby has been running a flight school for forty-six years, teaching people how to fly small airplanes. It's quite a feat. Even more so when you consider that she didn't start the school until she was in her forties.

Ruby oversees all aspects of the flight school, from accounting to maintenance to schedules. "I'll never retire," Ruby says. "I enjoy my work too much. And I haven't found any of it hard."

When she got her pilot's license, there weren't a lot of women in the air. "It just wasn't something women were expected to do," she recalls. "You got a lot of strange looks from the other pilots."

Still, she loved flying. "It's hard to explain why it's so much fun," she says. "You're up there by yourself, and it's quiet and peaceful. On a stressful day I could just go up in the air. It clears everything up. It's relaxing.

"It becomes second nature. It's a beautiful thing, a totally different world."

Though she's long since given up piloting, she still gets a thrill from watching the next generation learn how to fly: "It's like they are taking me up there with them."

People over age fifty were two times less likely to be proactive in response to periods of high stress in their lives than were people under age forty.

Simons 2002

26

The Best Life Needs No Trophy

It seems almost everything is competitive. People compete in an amazing array of contexts—from the job, to the home, to just about any arena you can imagine. For an example of how out of hand our competitiveness has become, just think about the fact that there are people today who make a living in competitive eating tournaments. One of the challenges of pursuing a satisfying life is that there is simply no competition. You will never live a better life because of the failure of another, nor a worse life for someone else's success. See your satisfaction in personal terms; your choices need not be justified to anyone or by anyone.

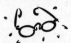

Paul has been swimming for more than seven decades. He has set records in his age group and won so many races that he's been inducted into the International Swimming Hall of Fame. But he's never had more fun in the pool than with the swimming club he helped found.

"Most swimming clubs are focused on training for specific competitions. Everything is competitive. We wanted more from a club than training, exercise, and an occasional race," Paul explains. "We wanted to create a friendly atmosphere for people who wanted to share their common love for swimming. Basically, we wanted to have fun, make friends, maintain good health, and improve as swimmers."

Doris has been swimming with the club for two years and can't tell you what her best time is, or her average time. "Swimming with the club has helped me to improve my stroke, but I really don't care how fast anybody swims," Doris says. "I don't even care how fast I swim, even though I swim three to four miles a week. It is good for my circulation, and it makes me feel good."

"These are the greatest people in the world," Paul adds. "My life is more fun now. That is what I wanted when we started, and I have it."

Men and women over forty who had above-average feelings of well-being were four times less likely to weigh their happiness and success against those of others.

Dube, Jodoin, and Kairouz 1998

27

The Future Can Be Brighter Than the Past

In most things, we've taught ourselves to see tomorrow as an extension of today. Things that are true now will continue to be true: The sun will rise in the east. Autumn will follow summer. But we are not limited in our happiness by the patterns we set yesterday. Our happiness is the product not just of our life experiences, but of our perspectives on them. Yesterday does not set the limit on our happiness today or tomorrow.

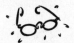

Mae saw the end of the nineteenth century, experienced every day of the twentieth century, and then welcomed the twenty-first century.

Mae has long since outlived her many friends and nearly all of her family. But her perspective on that is clear: "Always look forward, never back.

"When I get up in the morning, it's a blessing to have been given the chance to see another day. And I think that it just might be a good one."

Mae thinks people, whether they are old enough to remember when Woodrow Wilson was president or are too young to remember life before cell phones, should focus on all the possibilities of today.

"Enjoy what you have today," she advises. "Try to like the people around you and be good to them. Be kind and lend a helping hand. Try new things. Most of all, enjoy yourself, and remember that it's always better to laugh than to cry."

Two-thirds of those who characterized their experiences in childhood and young adulthood as unhappy reported that their lives in their fifties and beyond were happy.

Freeman, Templer, and Hill 1999

28

Stay in Control

Your life is the consequence of your decisions. Regardless of your life situation, you have to see that your decisions matter. Though embracing this view means accepting accountability and responsibility for your life—heavy burdens indeed—the most important thing that accompanies this belief is freedom.

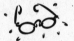

Rudy has spent four decades mentoring high school students as a teacher, counselor, and coach.

"The number one thing I tell kids—and it doesn't matter what context we're talking about—is that their decisions matter," Rudy says. "You don't want to study; that decision matters. You go out when you should be home; that decision matters. You goof off during practice instead of working hard; that decision matters.

"You have to be able to see cause and effect. Otherwise, even if you want the right effect, you won't know how to cause it."

Rudy has seen former students improve in school, head off to college, and succeed in careers. He says there is no better tribute to his personal belief that decisions matter than his former students' testimonials that they wouldn't be where they are today without him.

In eight out of ten people surveyed in one study, the feeling that their lives were beyond their control reduced their likelihood of life satisfaction by 40 percent and contributed to feelings of despondency.

Nair 2000

29

See Beyond You

Be open. Be welcoming. Be the person who wants other people around. Engage yourself in the lives of others, and you will see great rewards with minimal costs.

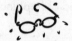

They had no illusions about being interesting. "We thought, 'Why not be up-front about it?'" Louis says. So they named their organization the Dull Men's Club.

This group of Massachusetts men meets once a month to discuss topics such as the migratory patterns of the hummingbird, the art of napping, and what they refer to as "Newton's law of inertia" (or, as club members sometimes call it, "the law that states that when you put a dull man in a seat, he stays there."). From the assigned topic, the men often veer into discussions of the world and of their lives.

Louis was inspired to try to bring people together after an experience he had on a ferry. Unexpectedly alone for the ride, he dreaded spending the two hours with nothing to occupy his time. Forced to approach a half-full table to find a seat, he began a conversation.

"I didn't spend a quiet moment in that two hours," Louis says. "We were all trading stories." Louis says that when he got off the boat, he felt like a new man. "I wanted to try to do that for some of the men in town," he adds.

Louis says that the Dull Men's Club serves a vital function for its members because so many men don't talk much about their problems. Instead, they internalize things, which he says ends up making them feel more alone. "Men tend to isolate more," Louis says. "To get them out of the house and talking is not an easy task."

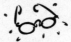

Research on retirees found that the most valuable personality trait in predicting happiness was extroversion—a tendency to seek company and to associate with others—which increased the likelihood of happiness by 47 percent.

Francis and Bolger 1997

30

Transitions Can Be Both Happy and Sad

We like to see things in clear terms: Hot is the opposite of cold. Small is the opposite of big. Happy is the opposite of sad. But our emotional lives are more complicated than that. We can be both happy and sad at the thought of transitions in our lives. Understanding this allows us to see sadness not as the enemy of happiness but as a natural part of our reaction to life.

These days, Phil knows he had a very rare job experience: thirty years for one employer.

Shivering through a New York winter, Phil set out for Florida with visions of palm trees and sea breezes. He heard that the phone company was hiring and put in an application. After hours of aptitude tests, he was hired and sent off to phone-installer classes.

"From the first day on the job I was comfortable with what I was doing. I liked it," Phil says. "I liked going out in a truck in the morning and being on the road and doing the work. I knew within a couple of days on the job that I would never want to do anything else."

Over the years, the technology changed and the job got a bit more complex. But, he says, "I liked the challenge. You had to learn something new every year."

Now, thirty years later, Phil is retired. He takes care of the house and cooks for himself and his wife. He plays endless rounds of golf at a course that allows him to play free in exchange for his occasionally helping out.

And how does it feel? "I feel like a kid again," he says. "Sometimes I'm the kid who just got out of school for the summer, and sometimes I'm the kid whose friends are all away at camp."

Researchers found that major life changes could produce strong simultaneous feelings of happiness and sadness.

Larsen, McGraw, and Cacioppo 2001

31

Embrace Challenges

There are many things we wish to do—from changing a tire to changing our lives—that we avoid because we are afraid of failure. We fear the direct evidence of our weakness, so we don't even bother to try. Ironically, our lack of effort is our true weakness. You are stronger and more capable than you can possibly know. When events occur and strength is demanded of you, you will be strong. Realize that you need not wait for events to call. You can demand strength of yourself right now.

Sydney Besthoff was born into the drugstore business. His grandfather was the cofounder of K&B, a modest chain of New Orleans–area drugstores. As a young man, Sydney was given an ever-shifting job in the business, starting as an assistant manager in one store, then moving on to purchasing, then finance, then personnel, then store operations.

After more than a decade of working in almost every job in the business, Sydney was promoted to running the company. In the ensuing decades, he took a collection of 15 stores and expanded it into one of the largest drugstore companies in the United States.

But after more than fifteen years of running the company, and more than twenty-five years of working for it, everything Sydney had ever done came under attack. Family members, including his sisters and his parents, sued him, claiming that he had cheated them out of their share of the company's profits. "It was a very upsetting time," Sydney says.

"It was a cataclysmic blow to him," his wife, Walda, adds. "He thought he was being a good son and a good brother. And when his family turned on him, it was heartbreaking for him. He felt betrayed."

But Sydney did not crumble under the strain of legal action and the animosity of his loved ones. He explained to them that his strategy of focusing on growth ahead of profits would be necessary until the company was big enough to compete with the major chains. His family either did not approve or did not believe him. "I told them to wait, that they would be very pleased in the end," he says.

Instead, they insisted on pursuing their legal actions, and Sydney ended up paying his relatives for their share of the business. "Anyone else might have folded, lost everything. Sydney found the strength to keep on going," Walda says. And in the end, the company continued expanding and succeeding until Sydney sold it to a larger rival chain.

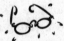

Studies of victims of traumatic events—such as people who lost their homes to natural disasters—found that those who had suffered the most loss of comfort were actually calmer and more resolute than those who had suffered some inconvenience but minimal loss.

Ikeuchi and Fujihara 2000

32

Get Away from It All

In every life there should be regular moments of awe. For most of us, our homes and communities may meet our usual needs, but they seldom inspire us. Take time on a regular basis to put yourself in a completely natural setting. Leave the city or the suburbs, and see the forest and the trees.

Carole grew up on a busy street in the middle of Richmond, Virginia. "All day long, something would be happening," she recalls. Across the street was the bus depot, where all the buses returned at the end of the day and started up again at the beginning of the next. And, as if that wasn't enough activity, Carole lived among six siblings and all the attendant chaos.

When she was seven, her family took a trip to Grayson County, in the Virginia countryside. "It was like I landed on another planet," Carole says. "Everything was green, everything was alive and beautiful, and the sky was so big, it looked like it went on forever. And as far as you could see, no other people."

Carole never forgot that trip. Five decades later she returned to Grayson County and bought some land and a century-old house. "We thought we were going to tear it down and build something new," she says. "But then I thought, 'This house belongs here.'"

The house looks out over a field and a glistening creek. "I like to listen to the creek. In fact, it's about the only sound out there most times," Carole says.

At first, she had to learn to sleep in such a quiet place. But the payoff was in the morning. "You wake up and the birds are singing," she says. "It's so peaceful."

People who regularly experienced nature were 9 percent less likely to report feeling unsatisfied with their lives.

Gerdtham and Johannesson 2001

33

Live Beyond Your Family Model

Most of us imagine that as we age, everything becomes easier—that we will have experience and wisdom to guide us. But the truth is that for all the years we've lived, we've never before been fifty, or sixty—or retired. We tend to fall back on examples we are familiar with, especially models from within our family. But we don't need to limit ourselves to repeating the lifestyles we observed there. Approach life with a full awareness of the possibilities that are yours.

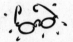

As she contemplates retirement, Joan thinks of the many changes she has seen in her everyday life. And she knows she has to find a new path for herself, one that is different from the path her parents and grandparents took. "When I was in school, we had just started into the space age. Television was just starting out. We couldn't have imagined all the ways life would be different today. But I tend to be an optimist about a lot of things," she says. "We know better how to treat our bodies, and hopefully the planet, too."

When her parents retired, they stopped working completely. "They just started an entirely new life," she says, "and they really weren't prepared for it. They thought it would be like an endless vacation, or at least that's what they said. But they always looked like the vacation never started."

Instead of leaving work entirely, Joan has created a schedule that will gradually decrease her hours until she has part-time status. "I'm trying to learn from some of the mistakes I've seen people make, and hopefully my daughter will learn something from me, too," she says.

Joan's daughter has already stepped down a different path. "I've never left the country, not even once," Joan says. "My daughter's living in Switzerland. Can you imagine that?"

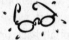

Surveys of people over fifty reveal that 66 percent took a family member's experience into account as they thought about their retirement plans.

Weigel, Bennett, and Ballard-Reisch 2003

34

Life Gets Easier

Some parts of life—mowing the lawn, moving furniture, and so on—get harder and harder as we age. But life itself tends to get easier. As we age, we tend to find deeper meaning in the things that truly matter to us. Take comfort in the thought that the most important things are getting easier, not harder.

"The great misconception younger people have is that older people are unhappy because of their age or that they spend their time wishing they were younger," says Jon Harris, a gerontologist who is old enough now to include himself among his subjects of study.

"Instead," Jon says, "age is really a blurry indicator of life quality.

"Physically, you can live your life in such a way that your body is in effect younger than your age. And you can live your life in such a way that your body is older than your age. So there is no way you should feel at any particular age. It varies tremendously.

"Mentally, you can see that older folks have a capacity to demonstrate resilience and recover from difficulties in their lives that is equal to or most often exceeds that of younger people. There is an inner fortitude that comes with experience, that comes with perspective. And it is one of the talents of our more senior citizens."

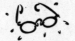

Research on people over sixty revealed that six in ten showed increased optimism, less stress, and an increased appreciation of others as they got older.

Kinnier et al. 2001

35

Volunteer for Yourself

Volunteering for a cause you care about is not only a great benefit to others but also a great benefit to yourself. Volunteering demonstrates our own humanity to us, and it offers us a wonderful opportunity for cultivating feelings of connection to our community. Give of yourself to others because it is the greatest gift you can give to yourself.

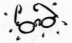

Frank has a simple explanation for the finding that at least half of people over age fifty spend part of their week volunteering: "There's only so much golf you can play. That's a fact."

But there's a more serious reason Frank spends two days a week volunteering in the Consumer Protection Division of the Maryland attorney general's office: "Number one, it helps people. Number two, it helps me."

Frank deals with citizens who have had consumer disputes with area companies. Frank takes their information and tries to work out an agreement between the customer and the company. "Some of these folks have spent literally everything they have on some-thing they really need—maybe a car, maybe a refrigerator," Frank explains. "Then it doesn't work, and the seller says, 'Tough.' Or they've signed on for a service they didn't really understand and can't really afford. Now they want to cancel but are told they can't. We step in, try to figure out the basic facts, and try to move the situation forward."

It's not only helping people but also working with his mind that Frank values in the experiences. "It keeps me sharp," he says. "Getting all the details straight. Figuring out the steps to follow. It's a new challenge every time."

Despite the complexities of the task, Frank is no lawyer. He thinks people imagine they have to be experts to volunteer in his office. "We're looking for people with common sense and life experience here," Frank says. "If you have that, you could be a valuable volunteer almost anywhere."

Researchers have found that volunteering improves life satisfaction across the generations. Notably, the effect is greatest among those over age sixty, who enjoy 72 percent greater life satisfaction and 54 percent more positive feelings about themselves when they volunteer.

Van Willigan 2000

36

Never Give Up

There are stories we hear about people becoming an overnight success. Of course, it often took them decades of anonymous hard work to get there. Regardless, success never stops satisfying. Far from losing its power, success late in life is every bit as satisfying as success at a younger age.

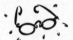

Frank McCourt taught writing and literature to New York City high school students. He dabbled in writing himself. But he'd never published anything.

Central to who he was as a person was his experience growing up within his family in his small Irish hometown. It was a life of great sadness, surrounded by poverty and alcoholism, but it was not without its humor and absurdity. Retired from the classroom, Frank committed himself to putting that story on paper.

The result was *Angela's Ashes,* a book that won millions of readers and the Pulitzer Prize.

Frank leaped from total obscurity to international fame.

"It's all a big surprise to me, all a big adventure. And I don't know where I'm going. It's a series of shocks," he says.

"But it hasn't changed me in any fundamental way," he adds. "I don't have time to get a bloated ego. God knows, I've taken time off, gone into a corner and said, 'OK, ego: bloat!' And it won't."

The capacity to continue trying despite repeated setbacks was associated with a more optimistic outlook on life in 31 percent of people studied, and with greater life satisfaction in 42 percent of them.

Meulemann 2001

37

Get Out of the Car

Driving is so much a part of most people's lives that they forget the incredible burden it can be. Few tasks require such a commitment to comprehensive concentration as we pay attention not only to what we're doing but to what every other driver is doing, not to mention walkers and anything else that might enter our path. Anything you can do to cut down on your daily driving time—car-pooling, relocating, planning your route—will reduce the amount of negative time in your day and free up positive time.

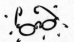

During a year the average Los Angeles resident spends the equivalent of three months' worth of workdays just driving to work. Two weeks of that time are spent sitting in stop-and-go traffic.

"Driving is one of the great eaters of time in our society," says sociologist Walter Rose. "Many of us see the freedom of driving—of going where you want, when you want—but we overlook the very real costs.

"Driving time is not time that's particularly good for anything else. If you are walking or riding a bicycle, you are getting exercise.

If you are taking a bus or train, you can read or work. If you are driving, you are just driving. At least that's all you should be doing if you want to be safe."

Professor Rose says that people often make the decision to live farther from their jobs because they think it's going to lead to a better use of their time. "They see the freedom of being right where they want to be on a Saturday morning. But they need to consider where they're going to be Monday through Friday morning, too—which is stuck in traffic."

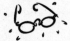

Every additional ten miles in a daily commute increases stress levels by 5 percent.

Lucas and Heady 2002

38

Don't Gamble Your Future

In the ads, everyone who places a bet or buys a lottery ticket is a winner. In reality, all forms of gambling are based on the inevitability of loss. More important, though gambling can be entertaining, it tends to make us feel out of control, not only of the outcome of a wager, but of our lives as well.

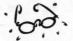

Susan Gaines conducts research on gambling and people who gamble. She says the picture of the problem gambler is changing rapidly to include more women and more people of middle age and older. And the reason, she says, is clear: "It's a process that starts with scratch-off lottery tickets and bingo and then progresses to slot machines. Casinos are going out of their way to reach new customers, including women over fifty."

Susan says that growth within the gambling industry largely depends on finding new customers. "Casinos work hard to offer some characteristics very important for individuals who in the past would not gamble," she says. Slot machines and other electronic gambling devices offer what Susan says is a welcoming environment to the novice gambler and to women in particular. "It's a relatively cheap way to begin playing. It feels physically safe and attractive," she says. "For a lot of people, it's an antidote to boredom.

"New gamblers don't like to be aggressive or carry on a conversation with a blackjack dealer. They want to get off by themselves, be safe, and sit down with nobody bothering them. It's real easy for someone to get sucked in to slot machines. They're mesmerizing. You lose all consciousness of the value of money.

"Nobody chooses to develop a gambling problem, of course. But you need to watch out, especially if you begin to shield others from your gambling plans. It's the first step toward losing control."

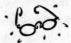

Adults over sixty who regularly gamble are 17 percent less likely to feel satisfied with their lives and 9 percent more likely to feel that their lives are not within their control.

Winslow 2001

39

Find a Physician You Like

It may sound superficial, but one of the most important things we need in a doctor is a pleasant personality. We need to have a good feeling about our doctors. For all their training and ability, if we feel disconnected from them, if we feel they think of us as a just another widget, we are less likely to seek their help and listen to their advice.

Don was having trouble getting through to his doctor. He called several times and left messages but didn't hear back. He debated whether he should start looking for a new doctor but also wondered whether perhaps he was overreacting.

When Don finally received an appointment, he arrived to find that his doctor was overbooked. After waiting all morning, Don finally was able to see his doctor, but for less than ten minutes.

So Don decided to do a little research. He was shocked to find out that the doctors' own association, the American Medical Association, reported that as many as a quarter of patients switch doctors because of problems communicating with their doctors.

"I began to understand that this wasn't just me," Don says. "Whether it seems no one is listening when you have an appointment, or you can't get through to make an appointment, when you can't communicate with your doctor, you feel like you don't matter."

Don found that the doctors' association offered various helpful hints for physicians in dealing with the personal side of the job. "It said that the personal side, how they treat people, is where trust comes from," Don says. "Without that trust, all the scientific knowledge in the world doesn't do the patient much good."

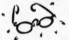

People who rated their physician as friendly were two times more likely to seek medical attention at the first sign of distress and were three times more likely to follow medical instructions than were those who rated their doctors as unfriendly.

Auerbach, Penberthy, and Kiesler 2004

40

Who You Are Is Not Just What You Do

The first question people ask when they meet someone is usually "What do you do?" We label people by their work before we know any other fact about them. Of course, work is part of who we are. It is part of what we know, how we spend our time, and what we care about. But to base our notion of a person, especially ourselves, on work is to miss the essence of who we are and of who we will be after work is over.

Gary is on a crusade to advance small talk beyond its current boundaries. "It's time to dismiss, 'How are you?'" he says. "When someone asks you that question, the only socially acceptable response, regardless of the truth, is 'Good. Yourself?' Anyone who responds honestly to 'How are you?' is marked as some kind of social misfit."

Gary is not a big fan of the initial question we often ask when meeting new people, either. "When you ask, 'What do you do?' before anything else, immediately I become my response, regardless of any other fact about me," says Gary. "There's a context where what you do may be relevant. But there are many more situations where it's not. If I say, 'I'm a plumber,' then I'm a plumber. Even if I later reveal I'm a socialist and play the flute, which may tell you a lot more about me than what I do, I'll still just be the plumber who happens to be a flute-playing socialist."

In this respect, Gary admires the way children interact. "Have you ever heard a child ask a question if they didn't care about the answer?" Gary asks. "No. Children ask questions because they actually are curious about something. That's why you never hear children ask, 'How are you?' And since children don't have jobs, they don't tend to ask, 'What do you do?' And yet, they somehow seem to manage to meet each other and make friends."

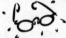

Those who based their identities strongly on their work were 24 percent less likely to maintain life satisfaction through their fifties and into retirement.

Reitzes and Mutran 2002

41

Foundations Shift, but Life Stands

There will be challenges and changes, to be sure. But the unspoken truth is that you are getting stronger, not weaker. Your resilience will see you through the good and the bad, and your capacity for making a life filled with happiness will persist.

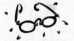

Henry was living off his investment earnings from the stock market. He lived well and was quick with advice for friends and family on how they, too, could make money on the market.

Then his investments started slowly shrinking. His broker suggested he take some of his assets out of the stock market, saying the market was too volatile and that a person of Henry's age shouldn't take such risks. But Henry was convinced he had made good choices. Says Henry, "I said to the broker, 'I want you to stay out of my way. I do my own research. I buy when I want to buy. I sell when I want to sell.'" Henry didn't want to sell. He waited for the market to pick up again.

But it didn't. Small losses became larger losses. And larger losses eventually swallowed his entire portfolio.

Henry sold his car. He downsized his home. And now he wears a coat indoors during the winter so that he can set the thermostat lower and sits in front of a single fan in the summer so that he can leave the air conditioner off. "That worked out to fifty dollars a month off my electric bill," he says.

Gone, too, are the daily trips to the local diner for breakfast. "I'm saving four dollars a day by not going there to eat," he points out.

Henry considers his situation his own doing. "The greed in me didn't want to see it," he says. "I knew I wasn't supposed to put all my eggs in one basket. But I did it anyway."

Despite it all, he maintains his sense of humor. When someone says he lost his shirt in the market, Henry says, "I lost more than my shirt. I lost my socks, my shoes, my hat." But Henry learned something about himself: "I'm a heck of a lot more resilient than I thought I was."

Experiences such as seeing one's income decline or one's family separate, which are related to low life satisfaction in younger people, have less effect on the long-term happiness of people in their fifties and beyond.

Diener and Suh 1998

42

Share What You Know

There are things you know that other people would love to know and that you would enjoy sharing. Seek the opportunity to share what you know, and you will be rewarded with an opportunity to focus your attention on your abilities and accomplishments. And you will have helped someone in the process.

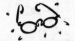

The caller might say they are from the credit-card company, or a utility, or a store. They will say there has been a problem, maybe some information has been lost, or the computer malfunctioned. Can you just confirm some information on your credit file one more time?

As Rick explains to people in his California hometown, such calls are scams that allow thieves to find out crucial information so they can ultimately get credit in your name. "These companies already have all your information," Rick says. "And if they didn't, they wouldn't call and ask you for it.

"Another popular scam involves an offer from a stranger. The stranger offers a check for a large sum of money. In exchange for your help in cashing the check, you will be able to keep 25 percent of the money. The check—or, in some cases, the wire deposit—is phony. The point of the offer is to get you to reveal your bank-account number, and when you do you'll find that instead of depositing a big check, somebody has written a big check against your account."

Rick serves as a volunteer, helping his local police department keep people informed about some of the sneakiest crimes out there. "Identity-theft issues are major, because you can be hurt without even knowing it," he says. "All your assets—your bank account, your credit cards, your home—could be targeted."

Rick gives talks to groups and offers tips not only about the latest scams but about how to protect yourself and what to do if your identity is stolen. "The most important thing is to be proactive," Rick says. "Anyone who gets access to your credit is going to try to create as much damage as they can as fast as possible."

Researchers studying people in their sixties have found that those who said they were in a mentoring-type relationship were 29 percent more likely to see meaning in their lives.

Van Handel Eagles 1999

43

Discuss Your Worries, Then Don't Dwell on Them

Some people keep their fears bottled up and just soldier on. Others are so enmeshed in their worries that they can think and speak of little else. Neither of these extremes is healthy. Voice your concerns to those you are closest to, because you will feel better opening up, you will feel closer to them, and often your problems will seem smaller when you get another person's perspective. But do not live within your problems as if it is they, not you, who exist.

"You don't spend your life farming without more worries than you can count," says Gus, who along with his wife, Emma, has spent more than four decades farming.

All year round there are endless chores and constant worries about all the things that must go right for the crops to flourish.

Each year is a careful balance in which the uncertain crop yields must be enough to pay the certain debts, the mortgage on the land, and the payments on the tractors and combines. During some rough years, Gus says, "we came so close to losing this farm so many times, it was unbelievable."

And if that's not enough, each year more of the farms in their area have been sold to housing developers—not only threatening a way of life but encouraging all the agriculture-related businesses that Gus relies upon to close up or move away.

Gus and Emma talk about the problems on the farm and reassure each other that even with the struggles, they are exactly where they want to be. "This is all we've ever wanted," Gus says. "To farm a nice piece of land, to raise a family. This has been my life, and what more can you ask for?"

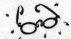

Those who felt comfortable discussing their worries with a close friend or relative were 11 percent less likely to feel overwhelmed by their concerns.

Gross and Simmons 2002

44

It All Looks Better over Time

The past never changes. Few things are more concrete and obvious than that. Yet, what we make of the past changes all the time. The good and the bad, the lessons and the mistakes, are subject to constant revision. Understand that we all have a tendency to rewrite our personal past, often smoothing out some of the rough edges to make the past look unrealistically good compared with today.

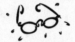

It used to be so much easier. People were nicer. It was quieter. Everything was cleaner. Life was just better.

Psychologist Kevin McNeil has heard variations on this theme from countless people. He studies the way people reflect on their past and finds that a certain creativity is often at work. "We look back at another time, and we immediately recognize that many things were very different," he says. "This gives us license almost to reimagine what life was like.

"Especially for those who are in a period of difficult transition, it is very tempting to take the past and hold it up as an example of what we wish for, all the while overlooking the struggles we went through then."

Professor McNeil recommends that people keep the positive memories of the past in mind, but not in a competitive or comparative way: "If you start measuring yesterday against today, you've taken something away from your life right now. Instead, if you stop to think about yesterday to celebrate it or to learn from it, then you've done something that contributes to today."

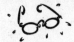

People interviewed over the course of several years became 2 percent more likely to report they had been generally happy in the past each time they were asked the question.

Field 1981

45

Keep Relationships on Level Ground

Feeling valued while valuing another is the surest sign of a strong relationship. Demonstrate in what you do and what you say that your relationship is balanced and meant for two people, not just one.

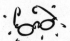

On their thirtieth wedding anniversary, Max and Sarah thought a lot about the journey they had been on together. "Two of our children were just beginning to plan weddings, and we wondered if there was anything we had learned that we could share with them," Sarah says.

Although they were in the midst of a celebration, their thoughts focused on some of the tough times. Sarah focused on Max's experience when he was laid off from a company that was downsizing. "It was awful for him," she recalls. "He had given a lot to the company and expected he would be with them for a long time. Some people, losing a job, would have crumbled from the blow to their ego. But Max never lost sight of his family and our love for him. And just as important, when he found work again, he never lost that appreciation and respect for the importance of his family relationships."

Max spoke of what it was like when he and Sarah were just starting out together. "At first, neither one of understood the other very well," he recalls. "There were so many frustrations. We had arguments over every silly thing in the book. It wasn't until we both began to see things from the other person's vantage point that we had any peace. We realized that it's not just the way you react to things, but the way you look at things. It's not just your view anymore. It shouldn't be, anyway. If it is, you're probably in trouble."

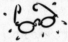

In long-term relationships, the feeling of equity was associated with a 29 percent greater likelihood of feelings of satisfaction with the relationship.

Donaghue and Fallon 2003

46

Adapt

There are milestones we know well and even enjoy. Events such as graduations and weddings are times of great upheaval that mark major transitions in our lives. Yet the reality is that a need to adapt to changing circumstances is never greater than in the second half of life. At an age when many are becoming more set in their ways, circumstances demand flexibility. Embrace change. It will be happening all around you, all the time. The more you can see change as an opportunity or at least as a challenge, the more satisfying you will find your life.

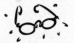

When George hears about someone retiring, he thinks, "That's nice. Talk to me when you've retired a third or fourth time."

George took early retirement from his career in engineering. At a more conventional age, he retired from his second career, in consulting. Bored at home, he soon took a job teaching, which he recently retired from so that he could have more freedom to travel. Lately, though, he's started doing some tutoring part-time.

"I figure, my granddaughter seems to graduate from something in school every year. She graduated from preschool, then from kindergarten; then she had some kind of ceremony when she played soccer. I'm trying to retire as many times as she graduates," George says.

Although he jokes about his experience, George thinks it's important for other people his age to be ready for change. "The nice way to look at it is: you have options," George says. "You can now ask yourself if you want to go to work or not. You can now ask yourself if you want to stay in this home or not. The harsh way to look at it is that all of a sudden the things you depended on may not be there anymore, or may not be right for you anymore."

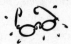

According to some studies, people in their sixties and older who were willing to be flexible about their lifestyle increased their life satisfaction by 38 percent.

Efklides, Kalaitzidou, Chankin 2003

47

Make Home Home

Your home must be a place of comfort for you. Invest in your community, whether that means the people in the house down the street or the person living across the hall. If you feel at home with them, you will feel at home at home.

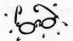

Florence moved to a North Carolina retirement community and discovered two things: she had no taste for the organized activities available in the community, and she had even less taste for sitting around alone.

"I was sitting here in the apartment by myself, and that is not healthy," Florence says. "I was getting depressed. I thought to myself, 'I've got to find something to do in the evenings.'" So she struck up a conversation with her next-door neighbor, talking about the things they liked to do. "We talked about books, and movies, and music, and art, and all kinds of things like that," she says.

And then they started planning small group trips to the movies. Each time they went out, their group grew slightly larger. "I was meeting at least one new person every time. And then people I was introduced to would later introduce me to others," Florence says.

Then she wondered if they should meet in the community clubhouse to talk about other things they might do together. The group set up a brief schedule of events with the idea that each occasion would be interesting but informal, with no need to sign up or pay anything. "Just come in if you want to," Florence explains.

Events have included debates, lectures, forums for local political candidates, and even book readings—not by authors, but by members of the group, who read from their favorite book.

"This group makes me feel at home here," Florence says. "This group bonds us together in a wonderful way."

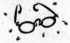

Positive feelings about neighbors have been found to be associated with a 16 percent greater life satisfaction and a 25 percent lower likelihood of experiencing feelings of loneliness.

Prezza et al. 2001

48

Don't Let Irritation Be Louder Than Joy

Which is more important, good or bad? Regardless of which you consider to be the right answer, bad is often a bigger part of our thoughts. The traffic jam that bogs down our day stays in our thoughts longer than the open road that sped us on our way. The rude clerk is memorable long after the nice clerk is forgotten. Remind yourself to see the good, to think about the good, to remember the good. The good is out there just as much as the bad, but we are often prone to miss it.

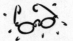

Katherine teaches a course on stress reduction. She sees people burdened with frustrations and tensions that overwhelm them. "You can get to a point where there's almost nothing else in your life," she says. "And by that point, your entire system, mental and physical, will be jeopardized."

Katherine asks her students to talk about some of the stressful moments they have faced that day. There's never a shortage of examples.

Katherine tells the class to think about all that they've heard from each other. "There is an infinite quantity of stress available to us if we choose to pursue it. The good news is, we don't have to take all this stress on," she says.

Katherine offers practical tips for her students to avoid compounding the worst moments of their day until it becomes their worst day. "First, take a deep breath," she advises. "Deep breathing helps calm us down. Second, watch your thoughts. Negative or fearful thoughts create more anxiety and stress, so when you start heading down that road, change the subject for yourself. Third, give yourself an alternative. Practice visualization, and think about what you like and what you want to happen."

Among those over fifty, the hassles of the day were three times more prominent in their thinking than the pleasant moments of the day.

Hart 1999

49

Geography Does Not Limit Family Life

Families confront geographic challenges all the time. Whether because of the next generation moving off to find their own lives or the parental generation moving away to fulfill dreams of a new phase of life, families must deal with distance. But feelings matter more than mile markers. Share your feelings and communicate often with family members regardless of location, and geography will not be a factor in your relationships.

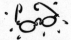

"When I was a little girl, if someone left to move to another state, you pretty much figured you would never see that person again," Janet says. "But now you could move to another country—heck, you could move to the moon—and you'd still be able to call and email."

Janet has grandchildren spread across three states. And though she loves to see them and spoil them, the most contact she has with them is by email. "I check my email all the time," she says. "And whenever I hear from one of them, I get a little charge inside."

Her grandchildren tell her about school, their activities, and the teams they play on. "I'm old enough to remember when people used to write letters. It's like we're doing that again. Except you receive them immediately, and you can answer right back," she says.

Janet took a computer course so she could master all the ins and outs of using the Internet and email. "In my circle of friends, I'm the only one who knows how to send and open pictures in email. I can do everything. I can send love to all my babies, all the time. It's the best thing going."

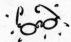

Increased geographic distance, whether caused by adult children moving away or by parents moving, did not reduce feelings of family closeness.

Glenn 1975

50

Vote

If you had a chance to help make a crucial decision, would you want to have a voice? If you had a chance to affect the future, would you act? The process of voting—from learning about the candidates to showing up on election day—is not only a crucial civic duty but also a means of connecting us to our community and giving us a feeling of personal responsibility.

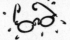

At a forum held at a South Dakota senior center, there were two things an audience of Democrats and Republicans could agree upon. The first, as Fred puts it, was "This campaign is a disgrace."

"Just disgusting," says Barbara. "The politicians are wasting a lot of time and money saying a lot of words, but they aren't telling us anything."

The complaints were about all the negative attacks their Senate candidates were sending out on television ads, radio ads, and mailings.

Just as upsetting as what was being said, for some, was what wasn't. "When will they have a moment to address the economy, roads, schools, the high cost of living, health care, housing? They never get to those because they are too busy calling each other names," Barbara says.

The other thing the people at the forum agreed upon was the importance of voting. "It's almost like they don't want us to vote, what with all these negative, nonsense ads. But I'll tell you what: they can't keep me out of the ballot box. Even if I have to vote 'None of the Above,' I'll be there," Fred says.

"I haven't missed a vote in forty-eight years," says Barbara. "It's too important to stay home. Staying home is like saying you don't care what happens to yourself or anyone else."

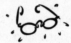

People who vote are 46 percent less likely to report feeling distrustful and dissatisfied with government and 8 percent more likely to report feeling satisfied with their lives.

Frey and Stutzer 2000

51

Forgive

We think of forgiveness as something we give to another person. But the burden of being angry and disappointed weighs us down, eating away at our relationships and bringing pain to our days. Forgiveness is not a sign of weakness any more than anger is a sign of strength. Try to forgive—if not for someone else, then for yourself.

"A grudge is not being able to get out of your mind some injustice you think somebody committed against you. Too many people are carrying them around," says psychologist Judy Lewis.

Regardless of the type of behavior that disappointed you, "for your own well-being, you need to get rid of the grudge," Professor Lewis says. "Forgiveness is absolutely essential if people are going to move forward in their lives.

"When you refuse to forgive, you have turned control of your emotional life over to the very person who has hurt you. Only by forgiving can you sever your emotional and psychological ties to the offense, so they lose the power to hurt you.

"There is also the self-interest of protecting your own health. A growing body of research on forgiveness suggests that forgiving lowers blood pressure, reduces stress and depression, and boosts the functioning of the immune system."

Ask yourself this question, Professor Lewis suggests: "Do you really value what that person did or said to such an extent that you are organizing your life around that person and sacrificing your own health?"

In order to forgive, you don't need to condone or excuse the inappropriate behavior of the person who offended you, she adds. "You forgive precisely because what they did was inappropriate. If it was appropriate," Professor Lewis asks, "what would there be to forgive?"

People with a higher tendency to forgive experience less stress and are 21 percent more likely to feel strong social connections.

Berry and Worthington 2001

52

Eat for Nutrition, Not for Compensation

When you water a plant, you give it whatever water it needs. You don't give it extra just on a whim. It should work the same with humans and food. But food for many is a tool for regulating their mood. Food as anything other than a source of nutrition transforms it from a requirement of life into a source of danger.

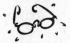

Jennifer is a nutritionist who specializes in working with people in their late fifties and older. "I see a lot of people who never really gave food a second thought. If they liked it, they ate it. If they didn't like it, they stayed away," she says. "Then they get to a point where they are concerned about their health or wish to get into better shape, and for the first time they consider how big a decision they have made by never deciding to eat right."

Jennifer says that although everybody would benefit from eating right, bad eating habits are a more serious concern for older people than for younger people: "As we age into our forties, fifties, and above, we lose bone density and our metabolism decreases. This means that what our body needs to thrive changes significantly as we get older."

Jennifer tells her clients that one of the more valuable things they can do is change how they eat. "People over age fifty should consider throwing out the idea of big sit-down meals and instead think about eating smaller meals more frequently throughout the day," she says. "Small portions throughout the day help us to maintain our energy level—instead of having it plunge and peak around our big meals. This also helps because making better use of the food energy we create means we burn more calories."

As for what to eat, Jennifer again emphasizes meeting the body's needs. "To keep their bones healthy, people should make sure they are getting the recommended daily dose of calcium and vitamin D," she advises, "and they should moderate their consumption of caffeine and soda. Drinking more water is an excellent alternative.

"The most important thing is for people to be aware of what they are doing and what they could be doing. A lot of folks don't mind making more healthy decisions if they know what they should be doing and why."

People with low life satisfaction were four times more likely to develop a habit of continuing to eat once their hunger was gone to compensate for depression.

Timmerman and Acton 2001

53

We're Happier Older Than Younger

The caricature of young people is that they are carefree and happy. The caricature of older people is that they are grumpy and serious. We think that getting older is inevitably a step away from joy, when actually the opposite is true. Aging by itself is no threat to happiness, and in fact older people are generally as happy as younger people, or even happier.

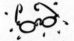

Sam approached his upcoming sixtieth birthday with dread: "I was imagining it was going to feel gloomy—like being sixty was a burden I would have to carry."

And the truth is, he did feel awful on his birthday, but not for the reason he thought he would. "Let's just say I may have picked the wrong day to try Thai food for the first time," he says.

Back on his feet the next day, Sam realized he didn't feel at all bad about being sixty. "It was like all this time I had been preparing for how bad things were going to be, and then I realized I didn't feel bad—I felt great," he says.

Sam decided to dedicate his upcoming year to visiting the many places in the country he'd always wanted to see, and to visiting as many relatives as he could.

"People say youth is wasted on the young," Sam says. "Well, I'm beginning to think that our golden years are wasted on the old. There's so much to do and so many options, if only we see them. We sometimes overlook, from a distance, how many pressures there are on young people to get their lives going in the right direction. By comparison, my friends and I have a pretty good thing going."

Studies comparing people over age sixty with those under age thirty-five found that those in the older group were 8 percent more likely to feel happy about their lives.

Mather and Carstensen 2003

54

Each Part of Life Must Function

A good job will make life satisfying no matter what life is like at home. A good life at home will make work satisfying no matter how hard it is. These are common ideas, but they are not true. Positive feelings from one part of our lives will not overcome difficulties in another. You must strive for satisfaction in every realm of your life that matters to you.

With a career path that led him down three very different directions and a family life that has at times been a great struggle, Larry has given a lot of thought to the balance of work and home life. "I've had times when I've worked too much and not paid enough attention to my family's needs," Larry recalls. "And I've had times when I was thinking about my family and not concentrating on my job.

"I read about an expert who said people were working longer hours just to stay away from their families. But how can that really work? Your family is part of who you are. Do you really think you can turn that off just because you're in an office somewhere?

"And it works the same the other way. If your job is dragging you down, you won't forget that burden when you are back home.

"Work and home life are pieces of us. If one's broken, we're broken. It's like with a car: three working tires do not make up for a fourth that is flat."

Among those over fifty, feelings about work had no value in predicting feelings about home life, and vice versa. Each set of feelings was independent and contributed separately to life satisfaction.

Hart 1999

55

See the Person, Not the Label

We know that we should think of others as individuals—each with their own needs, each with their own interests and abilities. But we fall into habits and assumptions that sort people out. Not only can this kind of thinking be a source of great conflict in our lives, but it also prevents us from seeing the capabilities of others, and even the capabilities of ourselves.

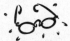

Rose doesn't spend a minute of the day outside her workplace without people making assumptions about her.

"If I bring my car in for service, they speak to me as if I've just stepped out of the stone age and can't possibly comprehend the basics of an engine," says Rose. Yet "in many ways I'm just like anyone else," adds the twenty-five-year teaching veteran who has spent even more years of her life as a nun.

"It makes the importance of looking within ourselves even more clear to me. We are so good at looking at the surface, at making assumptions. But those assumptions do not serve us when we're young, and they certainly do not serve us when we're older."

Rose learned early in the classroom that the poor students she encountered often floundered not because they were incapable but because people expected too little of them. "If you ask a person for the least they can offer, they generally will give just that to you," Rose says. "I dedicated myself to not operating based on expectations, based on what others may have concluded."

Especially as we get older, Rose says, preset expectations can close off potential friendships, sour relations within a family, and "make your life less than it could otherwise be."

People who were quick to apply stereotypes to others were 27 percent less likely to report that they were trusting of new people they met and 15 percent more likely to say they had trouble making new friends.

Amato et al. 2003

56

Laugh Your Way to Answers

Laughter is more than a smile and a fond memory. Laughter is fuel for hope. When we laugh, problems shrink and creativity flows. When we laugh, we see possibilities where we once saw only difficulties. Seek people and situations that make you laugh, and the parts of life that aren't funny will seem easier.

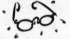

Long before he retired, he was depicting what he thought it would be like. In one scene, a group of spiders sits together on a front porch. One asks if he ever mentioned the time he was away from his web and a bug flew right into his mouth. One of the other spiders rolls his eyes, thinking to himself that he's heard that story a hundred times.

Gary Larson made up his own world of scheming cows, clever chickens, conversing insects, and nerdy scientists and turned it into a cartoon. His odd humor looked at life in unique ways through the eyes of humans, animals, and various sorts of monsters.

Starting with an occasional cartoon published in an obscure Seattle magazine, Gary's work captured people's interest and ultimately became the comic "The Far Side," carried in almost two thousand newspapers around the globe.

Gary believes his humor was a means to both amuse and offer some perspective. "There are worse ways to spend your time than having a laugh and maybe a thought every now and again," he says.

But he never sought the limelight, and with his cartoon following growing, he just walked away. His fear was that his work would lose its original humor.

Even though Gary is now out of the cartoon business, humor is still as important in his life. "Seeing the funny and the absurd makes for a good day," he says.

People who said they laughed a lot were 23 percent less likely to think there were obstacles in their lives that they could never overcome.

Olsson et al. 2002

57

Exercise

You know you are supposed to exercise. Every doctor will tell you that. What you might not know is that something as easy and pleasant as walking is a valuable exercise. What's more, exercise is as important for how you feel about yourself as it is for your health.

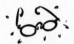

Tricia had never given serious thought to exercise except to imagine how awful it would be. "You see those people run by you on a summer day," she says. "They're drenched in sweat and look ready to pass out. I thought, 'If that's what it takes to be healthy, count me out.'"

But a trip to the doctor's office lead Tricia in a different direction. "He basically said I was an excellent candidate for just about everything you don't want to happen. And then he sent me to a fitness counselor," she recalls.

Tricia reluctantly followed her doctor's orders. She was surprised to learn how many different choices she had when it came to exercise. "You can exercise with a class full of people, if you need some kind of public aspect to get you to actually do something. Or you can exercise on your own, literally in your own living room," she adds.

Tricia started with a monitored walking program in which she would record her daily walks and periodically meet with her counselor. She found she wanted to do more and wound up signing up for a spinning class.

And now she says she never wants to stop. "It takes an effort to come here, but after exercising I feel 100 percent better," she says. "Once you get into the exercise routine, the mind and body basically require it."

Studies of people over fifty found that those who participated in a regular exercise program improved not only their health but their feelings of well-being by 39 percent.

Stacey, Kozma, and Stones 1985

58

Feed and Cultivate Friendships

We associate friendships with fun and goodwill. But friendships also take effort. We need to apply ourselves to the task of staying in contact and constantly tending to the foundations of old and new relationships. Though we are sometimes tempted to lose touch with friends because it is so easy to do, remember that each friendship we maintain adds purpose and joy to our lives.

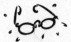

Emily and Pat were friends almost since the day they were born. "Our mothers were best friends. We were born just a few months apart, and from the start we would be in one another's home, playing with each other's toys," Pat says.

Growing up in New York City, they attended school together and were as close as sisters. After school, though, they drifted apart. They both got married and then went off, literally, in opposite directions as Emily settled on the East Coast and Pat on the West Coast. For many years they exchanged holiday cards and the occasional note, but they gradually fell out of each other's lives.

They'd had no contact for more than a decade when Pat had the idea of trying to track down her old friend on the Internet. "I didn't have her number or address anymore, and I had no idea where she might be," Pat recalls. "Imagine my surprise when I found an address for her and she was living only ten minutes away."

Pat wondered if she should call, but then couldn't stop herself. "After we talked, I felt like she just got back from summer camp," Pat says. "We just started right back from where we were before."

They see each other constantly, sharing meals and telling the stories of their lives. Still, Pat wishes she hadn't let the friendship fade away. "It's harder to keep close over time, and you can forget how much it means to you. I know this. I won't let it happen again," she says.

Having more close friendships was associated with a 19 percent greater life satisfaction and a 23 percent greater sense of optimism.

Richburg 1998

59

Communicate on Their Terms

Whether it's a personal conversation or a huge speech, the point of communication is to make ourselves understood. The desire to express ourselves in our own terms is strong and can lead us to lose sight of our audience. Don't think in terms of what you want to say; think in terms of what you want your listener to hear.

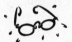

A roomful of people sit silent and still. They are hanging on every word Jay has to say.

Jay is speaking just above a whisper, describing how a young woman slowly gains the trust of a ferocious tiger. One day the woman plucks one of the tiger's whiskers and scampers off to give the whisker to a wizard who needs it to concoct a potion.

The audience gasps and groans with each twist of Jay's story.

Jay is part of a growing community of people who practice the art of storytelling. "Sharing stories is a very humanizing part of life," he says.

Jay doesn't read his stories from a book, nor are his audiences limited to children. Jay tells stories as a way of offering entertainment and of feeling connected to an audience.

And when he's not telling stories, he offers a class on how to tell stories. Jay emphasizes the importance of the audience's perspective. "Storytelling requires sincere eye contact and natural hand gestures to really keep a listener's attention," Jay explains. "You have to remember that holding their attention is the essence of the experience."

Jay believes people have the potential to be much better communicators than they realize. "Many people have a great capacity for storytelling and don't even know it," he says.

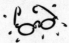

People who said they thought about things from their listeners' perspective were 48 percent more likely to be rated as effective in their communication efforts.

Chen and King 2002

60

Remember to Care for Yourself When Caring for Others

When we are a caregiver for a loved one, nearly all of our efforts are poured into that person's life and needs. It is truly a selfless act. But we must remember that to care for ourselves is not a selfish act. We have to make sure there is enough support in our lives to sustain the efforts we are making. Respecting your needs is the best way to continue offering care to someone else.

It happened right in front of her, in her own home. Brenda's brother Mark suffered a massive heart attack. He survived, barely, but his brain had been deprived of oxygen, and he had suffered brain damage.

At first Mark was placed in a group home. But he wandered away a number of times, once depositing himself on some railroad tracks frequently used by freight trains.

Brenda took her brother in because she wanted desperately to keep him safe, and she hoped a family environment would help him.

But every day is a struggle. Her brother keeps a random schedule, getting up at any time of the day or night, turning on lights and appliances as if preparing to head out for a job that doesn't exist. Each day Brenda must attempt to bring her brother back to reality, or close enough to reality to keep him safe and her household functioning.

"Mark's disability sometimes tempts one into thinking he can get better. He can do some chores around the house if I ask him. He can do the vacuuming, but you have to keep reminding him to keep going, because he forgets what he's doing while he's doing it," Brenda says. "Mark can remember Elvis Presley songs, because his long-term memory is pretty much intact, but he can't remember now or take in new information. He thinks there's nothing wrong with him."

Every time Brenda sought some kind of respite care, Mark rebelled. "We tried placing him in a center just for a few hours at a time, just for an afternoon. But he resisted," she says.

Brenda was ready to give up on the thought of as much as an afternoon alone, but counselors encouraged her to keep trying alternatives because, they said, no one can handle the burdens of providing constant care. "Finally we found a home health aide who Mark responded to without being threatened," Brenda says. "Now once a week she takes care of him for a few hours.

"Without her, I don't know what we would do."

Caregivers who relied upon the support of friends, family, or support groups to help them deal with the emotional burden of caregiving were 59 percent less likely to report feeling overwhelmed by their responsibilities than were those who faced caregiving alone.

Richardson and Sistler 1999

61

Be Careful Choosing Home Associations

Condominiums and other forms of community home owning are popular, and increasingly so for those heading into retirement. Give serious thought to the rules of any condominium you are buying into, though, and especially the enforcement techniques of the home owners' association. Community disputes are among the greatest sources of stress for many people, because there is literally no escape from them. Seek a community that not only fits your needs but fits your values as well.

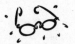

Bernadette is in her eighties and lives in a condominium with her Chihuahua, a dog so small it can fit in Bernadette's purse.

Officially, her condominium did not allow pets. But Bernadette didn't really think anyone would care about a tiny creature that did not make any noise and was never allowed outside on the condominium's common property.

For five years, Bernadette and her dog lived in her condominium without any problem.

Then one day a condominium board member saw the dog.

"No pets allowed," he said. Bernadette replied, "Get a life."

The condo association got an attorney and started proceedings to evict Bernadette. She held her ground, deciding that if she had to choose, she would rather lose her home than her companion.

"Just having her and petting her, it's very therapeutic," she says. "For older people, they have to have something to live for, something to take care of."

Many fellow residents jumped to her defense, signing a petition asking the board to stop its efforts against her and her dog.

Ultimately Bernadette received a reprieve with the help of her doctor, who said the dog was crucial to her well-being. But the experience soured Bernadette on her community. "Apparently around here it's rules first, people second, dogs third," she says.

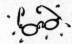

Participation in contentious organizations contributes to 24 percent increased stress levels and a reduced sense of satisfaction.

Bozeman et al. 2001

62

See Around Career Roadblocks

After enough time in a field, you become an expert. You know your job better than anyone else, and you know how things could be organized not only to make you work better but to make everyone around you work better. Often with this expertise, however, comes frustration, because there may not be any way for you to bring your vision into reality. Overcoming this frustration requires seeing another way around the problem. Find an outlet for your expertise, be it within your workplace or in some other setting.

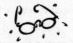

"Advertising is a strange line of work. It sits right at the intersection of creativity and commerce. If it's too much of one, it generally fails at being the other," Elliot says.

Elliot was good at what he did, but he often felt stifled by the limits of his work: "You can take something only so far before it's too new, too different, and then your idea will never make it through the internal steps and be presented to a client. And even if it did, the client would likely object."

Elliot saw this in his own career and also saw the frustration in his colleagues. "These are some of the most creative people you could imagine," he says, "but some of them felt like they were running a race with lead weights in their pockets, so that they could really never go as fast as they were capable."

Elliot realized he could not reinvent his company, much less the entire advertising industry. But he could provide a new outlet for bottled-up creativity.

Elliot opened a small gallery featuring all kinds of art and creative pieces. His first step was to invite his co-workers to bring him anything they might be secretly working on or have hidden in their garages and basements. He says, "They responded with paintings, drawings, photos, sculptures, jewelry, handmade furniture, and things you just can't describe.

"The art is nice, and the shop is even clearing a tiny profit. But the point of it is to feel all the way alive."

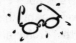

Research on veteran teachers found that 64 percent were burdened with significant frustration at administrators' lack of interest in their views. Those who overcame their frustration typically redirected their energies toward mentoring new professionals or finding an outlet for their expertise outside the school.

Clarke 1998

63

See a Kid, Be a Kid Again

Regardless of whether there are children in your family, there should be children in your life. Children not only bring an energy and a vitality to our day; they offer us a unique view of our life. Whether it's babysitting, coaching, or volunteering at your local school, find a way to involve yourself in a child's life, and you will feel like a kid again.

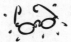

When Warren turned sixty-five, he started to wonder how much there was left to do.

Retired from a career in sales, Warren had seen his children move out long before. Apart from the occasional project around the home, there was little to do in the average day.

"You reach a point where you feel like you've accomplished what you set out to accomplish, or at least as much as you're ever likely to. And you look around and question not what comes next but whether there is a next," he says.

After taking a battery of tests inspired by a health scare, Warren came to learn he was in better health than he imagined. "Try as they might, the doctors couldn't find anything in me to worry about," he says.

Warren was ruminating over his future one day while taking a walk through a beachfront park. He saw a sign that read: Children Must Be Accompanied by an Adult.

He looked around and saw that there seemed to be an adult there with every child. Some of the adults he saw were building sand castles; others were playing ball. They were all smiling and having fun.

But there were plenty of adults there without a child. And he wondered if perhaps the people who wrote the sign got it backward. "Maybe it should say: Adults Must Be Accompanied by a Child," he muses.

Warren, taking the example to heart, went home and found the phone number for the local little league. Now he's an assistant coach for a team of seven- and-eight-year-old ballplayers. "I'll tell you this: I haven't had this much fun since I don't know when," Warren says.

Ninety-two percent of grandparents thought that the role of grandparenting had made their lives significantly more satisfying, in part because the contact made them feel young and excited.

Peterson 1999

64

Stretch

Do your body a favor, and stretch every day. It's not exciting. It seems like the kind of thing you would do before running a race. But it is important to give your body a stretch on a daily basis to help improve your circulation and to help prevent injuries.

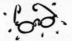

Sue learned the importance of stretching at an early age. "My father was a competitive gymnast. Of course, stretching was an absolute necessity for him before he began to subject his body to those kinds of strains," she says.

"Growing up, we had a miniature gym at home in the basement with rings, weights—the whole thing. He taught us from about as far back as I can remember the importance of stretching in a serious manner before you begin to exercise."

Sixty years later, stretching is still a part of Sue's daily routine: "First thing in the morning before breakfast, I do thirty minutes of stretching in my bedroom. I'm exhilarated afterward. You're aware of your body opening up, of being alive."

Sue thinks too few people appreciate the value of stretching. "It seems so passive, people doubt it does any good," she says. "But the parts of you that need stretching are not on the surface. The good it does is very real, even if you can't see it. A good stretching routine will not only help you heal if you get injured, it will help you avoid injury in the first place."

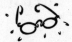

Studies of people over fifty found that those who stretched frequently were 11 percent more likely to say they felt healthy.

McAuley et al. 2000

65

Let Old Secrets Stay Secrets

Do you have to tell everything? No. There are many rewards for honesty and open communication. They are valuable foundations for a close and respectful relationship. But revealing long-held secrets can cause irreparable harm to a relationship, because time can serve to magnify the importance of the information. Share everything you feel you can, but realize there can be costs to sharing yesterday's secrets.

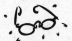

They consider themselves the ultimate interfaith couple. Laura is a minister at a conservative Christian church, and Robert is a minister at a Unitarian church that espouses no single religious foundation.

Laura and Robert have been married for twenty-two years, and when they are not leading church services, they work together, counseling couples. "When we say you don't have to agree on everything, we're living proof of that. We disagree on some of the most basic tenets of life. But at the same time we respect each other and each other's beliefs," says Laura.

Although they are open about their beliefs and their differing views, they tell other couples that that does not mean they share absolutely everything. "People get confused when they think that being open and honest means they say whatever pops into their head," Robert says. "That's not open and honest, that's communicating as a small child would. Open and honest is communicating what matters the most."

When someone is struggling with a past misdeed, Robert asks them to think about whether, if the shoe were on the other foot, they would want to know about it. "At first we all say yes, but given time, we come to question whether the pain of the information outweighs its value," he says.

For Laura and Robert, communication means they never shy way from serious discussions about their religious views, often leading to hours of debate. "But we never feel that everything we ever think, or everything we've ever done, has to be on the table," adds Laura.

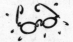

Studies of couples married for more than twenty years found that 62 percent thought that confessing a long-ago act was more dangerous than helpful.

Finkenauer and Hazam 2000

66

Listen to Your Favorite Music

A song is so much more than sound to us. It is a feeling, a memory, a new world, a trip back to an old world. Keep music in your life wherever you go.

Some have never played an instrument before in their lives. Others have been tinkering around with one for decades.

They have two things in common: they all love music, and they all are over fifty.

Members of the New Horizons Band, a national network of amateur musicians fifty and over, have organized more than one hundred chapters across the country.

"It's like a runner's high," says Peter, a retired doctor and a trumpet player. "Endorphins get released. You don't want to go to bed after we play."

Though many band members have to deal with some physical limitations, they all persevere. "With peripheral vision on the decline, it makes it harder for the musicians to watch the conductor," says Bob, who serves as a conductor for three Atlanta-area

New Horizons bands. Speaking with diplomacy, Bob says that such conditions make for "interesting times. Every performance is different." As one band member says of Bob, "He has a knack for telling you you're playing very badly without making you feel bad."

Senior players also enjoy advantages, Bob says: "They really want to play, and they have a lifetime of music in their heads. That's a fantastic resource to draw from."

"It's a great escape," Peter says. "When you're here, you can forget your other worries and troubles and get lost in the music."

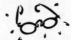

In studies of people in their sixties and older, all participants showed an improved mood and greater feelings of satisfaction when they were listening to their favorite music.

Burack, Jefferson, and Libow 2002

67

Practice Maintenance for Life

We don't buy a house or a car and expect it to stay in good working order over the years without regular upkeep and repairs. Yet we often think our relationships will keep going regardless of how we treat them. Give your relationships, whether friendships or family connections, regular attention and effort so that what you value will keep on being there for you.

"Everybody I know has a good friend, someone they were very close to, and then lost touch with. I was committed to trying to avoid that with these guys," says Tony by way of explanation for the twenty-second annual edition of the *Seventh Avenue News*.

As boys, Tony and his buddies grew up together in Brooklyn. "We all had plans. We were going to do this, see that, take over this," Tony recalls.

School, jobs, and the military quickly scattered the group. But Tony paid careful attention to his friends' addresses and would write them from time to time. "Soon the letters back and forth were filled with questions like 'Have you heard from Mickey?

What's he up to?' I decided that rather than our sharing the scattered information with each other one at a time, it made more sense to write it all down once."

Thus was born the *Seventh Avenue News,* filled with the goings-on of the buddies—their lives, their families, and their friendships.

Mickey says he's grateful for Tony's efforts: "Because of Tony, the people I considered friends for life when I was a boy really are friends for life. They have been a part of the major events of my life."

People who said that maintaining the health of their relationships was a priority were 22 percent more likely to find their social lives satisfying.

Weigel and Ballard-Reisch 1999

68

Call Town Hall

Your local government and countless nonprofit agencies exist to help you, whether you are looking for a tennis court to play on or need some advice on calculating your taxes. Often an area supports useful programs that few people are aware of. Call your city hall and ask about what's available locally. Not only will you benefit from the programs; you'll feel better about your community.

The town council of Wellington, Florida, decided that there was a disconnection between what the town had to offer seniors and what seniors knew about the town's programs. "You can work very hard to address the needs of a community, but if people don't know what you're doing, you can never really succeed," says Richard, who was hired to be the town's first senior-services coordinator.

Richard, working under Wellington's recreation department, found himself seeking to expand the town's offerings—which included an exercise program and a safe-driving course—while publicizing everything the department does.

He developed a wider series of courses and activities—and launched a magazine-style bulletin that brought together the town's offerings in one place and was sent to all residents. Richard made it a priority to create schedules further in advance, so that people could plan to attend. "Some of the courses we offer are ongoing," Richard explains, "and you are much more likely to attract people to a three-month program if they have some opportunity to plan for it."

Richard has seen the list of programs expand beyond the recreation-oriented services offered previously to include art and photography classes, current-events classes, and even events geared for grandparents and their grandchildren.

"We have a lot to offer," he says. "I just need to continue to seek out the areas where seniors are and let them know about us."

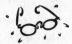

People who were aware of local and city programs for such things as transportation, recreation, and social support were 22 percent more likely to say they liked living in their communities.

Michalos and Zumbo 1999

69

Pay Attention to Nonverbal Communication

There is a big difference between talking to someone in person and talking over the phone. When we can see the person, we process not only what they say but everything about their appearance. As we age, we tend to be less attuned to the nonverbal cues that are presented to us. This means we lose much of what is being communicated, including hidden meanings and humor. If you want to know what someone is really saying, pay attention to more than simply what they say.

Harvey teaches a course on communication skills. "Half of what you are communicating does not come from what you are saying," Harvey maintains. He tells people that their eyes, their hands, and their posture are all telling a story, whether they consciously mean them to or not.

"As we get older, we increasingly become creatures of habit. Our walk is our walk, regardless of what it might look like. Our smiles and frowns are coming, regardless of whether they're appropriate," he says.

Harvey started with a focus on business communication but soon realized that communication habits were just as important in people's personal lives. "It may sound superficial to tell someone to think about their smile. It may sound superficial to tell someone to think about the way they sit in a chair," Harvey says. "But if the ultimate goal is to be understood, not misunderstood, you have to be aware of the messages you are sending."

At the same time, missing the cues others are sending is a sure contributor to conflict. "If you are not paying attention to the body language of the other person you are speaking with, you are likely to make more false assumptions about their thoughts and feelings," Harvey explains.

Harvey says it's all about understanding others and being understood. "If you don't know what a word means, you look it up. This is the same thing. If you don't realize what nonverbal messages are coming from you and to you, you need to find out," he says.

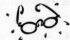

Researchers found that, compared with people in their twenties, people in their sixties were 27 percent less likely to correctly process nonverbal communication such as facial expressions.

Thompson, Aidinejad, and Ponte 2001

70

Wash the Dishes

Household chores are no one's idea of fun. But doing your share sends a message that you care about your home and want to fully participate in meeting all its needs. You can communicate respect with little acts as much as big.

Kathleen and Alf have been married for seventy years. The West Virginia couple have a simple recipe for a good relationship: she cooks; he cleans.

"You share what has to be done," Alf says. "It's a pretty simple thing. Nobody wants to have to do everything. And they shouldn't."

Kathleen credits her husband with understanding the importance of being a partner in all aspects of life. "He hasn't changed hardly any since we got married," she says. "He's always been willing to help me all he can."

Thinking about all the modern conveniences younger generations rely upon, Alf shakes his head: "And with all that, they just get more lazy."

Of course, they've had their disagreements. "You can't live with somebody seventy years and not have some spats. We made that vow, that we're going to make it," Kathleen says. "We have our ups and downs like everyone, but we never let it get that far to ever want to separate." Alf adds, "You've got to give and take. That's the only way to make it."

But beneath it all there has always been love and respect. "Show love and respect every day," Alf says. "Even if it's just cleaning up after dinner."

Willingness to consistently participate in household chores was associated with a 31 percent higher relationship satisfaction and a 15 percent higher life satisfaction.

Austrom et al. 2003

71

Be Open to a New View

There is no reason to start each day as if you must relearn everything and make up your mind again on every issue. That would be absurd. It would be equally absurd, however, to start each day as if there were nothing you might learn and no reason to reconsider anything you've decided. Be open to a new way of doing something or a new way of thinking about something.

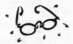

To John, novels were something you read because you were forced to. "Your English teacher tells you to read this five-hundred-page thing and write an essay. You trudge home carrying it, and every time you turn the page, you hope you've made it to the end," John recalls.

As an adult, John would read about people or places that interested him, but he had no interest in fiction. "It's all made up. What do I need that for?" he'd say.

One time he was a few minutes early picking up a friend from what turned out to be a book-club meeting. "I peek in, and all these people looked like they were having a blast. And all they were doing was talking about some book," he says.

John's friend told him he shouldn't dismiss the idea of enjoying novels just because he didn't care for them when he was fifteen. The book club was reading George Orwell's *1984* for its next monthly meeting, and his friend convinced John to give it a try.

"I picked it up, and I couldn't put it down," John says. "There is so much in there that applies to our society, our politics—I mean, about how they are today, in real life. I had a pen, and I was underlining different sections and writing little notes."

John attended the meeting and wound up in a heated discussion about the book and its implications. Though he didn't have any thoughts on which book the group should read next, he had definite plans to read their selection and attend their next meeting.

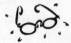

People over forty who could identify at least one change in their viewpoints or behavior in recent months were 8 percent more likely to feel hopeful about the future and 5 percent more likely to say they were generally in a good mood.

Grossbaum and Bates 2002

72

Love Evolves but Can Stay Strong

Any task that needs to be endlessly repeated is exhausting and intimidating. Having a strong relationship requires one loving and respectful day followed by another followed by another and on and on for beyond the foreseeable future. Although excitement may launch you on this journey, respect and concern will sustain you.

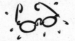

Roger and Connie have been married long enough to remember a time when people were expected to stay married forever. "There weren't many divorces," Connie says, "but that doesn't mean there were a lot of happy marriages, either.

"Most people have a certain role during a certain time in your life. Your parents are in the center of your life, but you grow up and leave. Your friends are in the center of your life, but then you get older and head in different directions. But your spouse is in the center of your life when you are just starting out, in the center of your life in the middle, in the center of your life at the end.

"What you don't know when you are starting out is that plain old-fashioned love is not enough. Everybody's in love when they get married, but if that were enough, there would be no divorce.

"How can you possibly keep your relationship strong over so many years? Is it hopeless? No, but you have to let it become a new relationship every now and then. It may start out all flowers and romance, but that can't last forever. It has to become a real friendship, a passionate friendship," Connie says.

"You need to enjoy the moments as they come," she adds. "Nothing stays the same forever, but good things can turn into other good things."

Married couples with high levels of mutual respect become 2 percent more likely to say their relationship is highly satisfying with each additional year they remain together.

Rosen-Grandon, Myers, and Hattie 2004

73

Use a Computer

With a computer, the world is literally at your fingertips. Whether it's to track down an obscure fact or to keep in touch with loved ones, computers give people a tool that helps them feel in control. You should make a computer a regular part of your life, because no matter what your interests are, a computer will help you access things that matter to you.

When the state of Maryland instituted a community-service requirement mandating that high school students spend some time volunteering for their community, Clarence had an idea.

Many of the seniors he knew were curious about computers but didn't know how to use them. High school students, Clarence reasoned, were probably the most expert computer users in town. He contacted school officials and asked if they had any students interested in fulfilling their community-service duties by teaching basic computer and Internet skills to seniors.

School officials were enthusiastic and sent over a group of teens. "Finding the seniors proved to be the difficult part. They were skeptical that they could learn something new," Clarence says.

But before long, a team of sixteen- and seventeen-year-old teachers were tutoring sixty-, seventy-, eighty-, and ninety-year-old students. The students lacked even the most basic knowledge of computers, but the teenage teachers patiently led them through the steps, starting with learning how to turn the machine on, and now the seniors are emailing, searching the Internet, and using software.

"I believe technology can be an enormous help in reducing isolation, particularly among the elderly. It can help people communicate, express themselves, expand their knowledge," says Clarence.

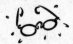

In people sixty and older, the personal use of computers for communication, information, and entertainment was associated with an 11 percent higher degree of life satisfaction.

Schiffman, Sherman, and Long 2003

74

The Youngest and Oldest Like Work the Least

You may not have very much in common right now with the twenty-year-old version of yourself or with your twenty-year-old relatives. But chances are you do have one thing in common: relatively less enjoyment in your work. Interest in work tends to peak in the forties because that is generally the time of greatest possibility in the workplace. Capture your interests, whether they can be used in the workplace or not, and see the larger world in which you can contribute.

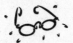

"From my perspective, you don't really want to be the new guy in the office or the old guy in the office," says Len, who was once the former and is now the latter.

"The new guy makes everybody else feel competent because he doesn't know how to do anything yet. He's useful mainly to go fetch heavy things from the storage closet. And there's always the underlying notion in everyone's head that if somebody has to go, it should be the new guy.

"The old guy makes everybody else feel competent because he doesn't know how to do anything anymore. He may know how to do things the old way, he may have even come up with the old way, but he hasn't kept up with any improvements in how things are done. And there's always the underlying notion in everyone's head that if somebody has to go, and the new guy turns out to be all right, then it should be the old guy."

To Len, being the new guy or the old guy requires you to see things beyond your routine. "You have to get out of that notion that life is what happens at work," he recommends. "Life is what happens when you are not at work.

"When you ask the question about meaning, about whether this is all there is, you need to answer no. Your energy is out there in the world. There is a need for your personal engagement in the things you care about."

Enjoyment of work is greatest among people in their mid-forties and is least among those in their twenties and sixties.

Hochwarter et al. 2001

75

Compromise What but Never Who

As we age, we get more set in our ways. It is a natural consequence of experience. Trying to get along with the people in our lives offers us a constant stream of opportunities for compromising to keep the peace in our social world. Of course, you should be open to seeing others' perspectives in general, and especially on things that are not crucial to you. But you should be willing to maintain your personal views on the things that matter most to you, because compromising who you are will prevent you from respecting yourself and enjoying your relationships.

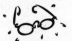

"You'd like to think that as you get older, I don't know if you get smarter, but at least you get a little wiser," Margaret says. "Maybe you don't know how to solve every problem or every disagreement, but you're supposed to understand better where these problems start, and maybe how to steer clear of them."

Margaret laments that within her family "fifty years of being sisters still doesn't seem to have taught us very much." Instead,

Margaret says, she and her two sisters are still having some of the same arguments they had when they were teenagers.

"The subjects may change a bit," she explains. "We're not arguing about boys or who gets to borrow the family car. But there's still this sense of jealousy, of an unstated pecking order in which each of us tends to see ourselves as first among the sisters."

Lately, Margaret has sought to try to figure out the difference between the disagreements that really don't matter and those that do. "I refuse, I absolutely refuse to have any variation of the 'who makes better pie' discussion ever again. I give up. I have nothing more to say in defense of my cooking," Margaret adds.

At the same time, Margaret says she simply can't bite her tongue when disagreements arise over the care of their mother: "This is too important to me. *Important* isn't even a strong enough word. How you treat your mother, especially when she is in need, is to me the definition of what kind of person you are."

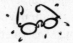

A willingness to compromise on trivial matters was associated with 62 percent more positive social relations, but a willingness to compromise on matters of values and personal vision was associated with 34 percent less life satisfaction.

Bargdill 1998

76

Your History Strengthens Your Future

Your personal history is not over. It is a part of you every day. The more you strengthen that history—by thinking about it, talking about it, writing about it—the more you will see the beauty of the life you've led and the possibilities of the life you are living.

Mary has lived through changes in everyday life she couldn't have dreamed of as a girl.

While she was growing up, just trying to get some light to see at night in her family's cabin was a terrible chore. "We had oil lamps," she recalls. "You had to fill them, trim the wicks, and you had to keep washing the globes, because they would get sooty."

Late in her teens, electricity finally came in. "All of a sudden, if you wanted light, you just turned it on," she says.

When she was a child, there was no indoor plumbing in the cabin, either. Mary, her parents, and her brothers and sisters used an outhouse set far back from their home. The thought of using the outhouse during the cold winter months still gives Mary chills. "You didn't stay long," she remembers. "You did what you went for and got out of there. When we finally got plumbing, I sure didn't miss the old way."

Though there was no shortage of hardships in her youth, Mary also enjoyed a close relationship with her parents, six sisters and two brothers, aunts and uncles, and grandparents.

It wasn't until she had a family of her own that Mary started writing about her childhood experiences. "My daughter said to me one time I had better put some of the stories down she was hearing from my parents and from me, because otherwise they would be lost forever," she explains.

Mary decided to sit down with pen and paper and see what would happen. "I was writing at first to give my children and grandchildren their history, but then I saw I was giving myself a history lesson, too. Sometimes you don't appreciate where you are until you take a good hard look at where you've been," Mary says.

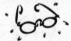

People who wrote about the history of their lives were 11 percent more likely to feel happy with their lives and 17 percent more likely to feel optimistic about the future.

Yamada 2000

77

Share Your Home

We generally think of opening our home to others as a sacrifice we make only until our children become adults. But sharing our home with others is good for us. Humans are social beings that depend on consistent contact with others. Sharing a home, whether in a family situation or with a friend or a roommate, creates a humanity in our lives that we cannot achieve on our own.

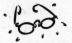

John has no patience with cooking. For him, preparing a meal gets no more complicated than pouring cereal and milk into a bowl. Guy was trying to find his way after a divorce left him unsure and alone.

Apart, these two fifty-something men found more struggle than hope in their days. But when Somerset County, New Jersey, started a program to help place county residents in home-sharing opportunities, John and Guy both thought for the first time about the possibility of having a roommate.

Introduced to each other by the program, neither man was convinced it was a good idea. "When you think about it, it sounds kind of strange. Who ever heard of moving in with someone you don't really know, and not because you have to but because you want to?" John asks.

But before long, both thought it was worth a try. Guy moved into John's home. They began by sharing chores but soon were sharing their stories. A friendship blossomed.

"Just because you live alone doesn't mean you always want to be alone," says John. "There is a need for friendship that never goes away. I'm grateful Guy and I could meet, because it has made life easier for both of us."

John admits there are compromises to be made: "It's a bit of an *Odd Couple* thing. He's neater than I am. But those are just idiosyncrasies. What matters is that you've got to give and take, and if you do, you have a friend."

People over fifty who shared their home with another person were 27 percent more likely to feel healthy, 32 percent more likely to feel optimistic about their lives, and 61 percent less likely to feel lonely.

Altus and Mathews 2000

78

Honor Your Spiritual Beliefs

Discomfort in our lives comes in many shapes and sizes, but the most pressing concerns are basic matters of life and death. We desire a life well lived and a death of grace. People with firmly held spiritual beliefs enjoy a strong sense of purpose in their lives and see death as another chapter in life. Let your spiritual beliefs guide you, not only to your ethic, but to your joy.

Robert has lived his personal and professional life around his religion. As a Presbyterian minister, he has mentored countless people through their lives, careers, and spiritual journeys.

Now Robert is making a major career transition of his own. With an eye toward his eventual retirement, he is sharing his church responsibilities with a young co-pastor, Brian. Robert and Brian alternate offering sermons and share the many small-group and personal counseling tasks that Robert has long built into his schedule.

Brian knows that many ministers could not accept the idea of sharing their workload, their position—their church—with anyone.

"I have been approached in the past to be a co-pastor in other situations, and I have declined because it really has to be a special pastor who would truly share the position. Robert has done that graciously," Brian says.

Robert sees the transition not as a threat to his ego but as a celebration of his faith. "My role is to help Brian help the congregation adjust from me to him and to his leadership," Robert says. "It keeps the momentum going, and it keeps people's interest high. This is not about the end of my role. It's about the importance of this church in the lives of all our congregants, including my own."

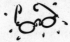

Regardless of which religion they subscribed to, those over fifty who said they had strong spiritual beliefs were 4 percent more likely to be happy.

Francis, Jones, and Wilcox 2000

79

Wear Many Hats

We use only a fraction of our powers. Most of us operate as if minimizing our efforts, whether intellectual or physical, were the ideal. When we maximally use our abilities to pursue our various interests, we maximize our capacity to live.

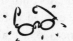

Sometimes, after William is introduced as an eminent historian, he rises to the podium to tell the audience about specific battles of the Civil War.

Other times he's introduced as a NASA engineer, and he discusses the next generation of spacecraft.

Still other times he's introduced as the Irish ambassador to the United States, and he analyzes our country's policy regarding Europe.

And occasionally he's introduced as a research biologist, and he discusses the struggle for life in Antarctica.

When William speaks, his comments are initially filled with jargon specific to the topic. "You can look around the room and see some people wondering if this is all going to be too deep for them to understand," William says.

But the real problem kicks in when someone asks a question. "Somebody once asked me how much time I spent in Antarctica doing my research. I said, 'Enough to know the polar bears by name,'" he recalls.

The questioner, looking puzzled, countered, "There aren't any polar bears in Antarctica. Polar bears live in the Arctic—the opposite end of the globe from Antarctica."

With a nod, William replied, "Is that right?" And then he came clean to his audience.

William, it turns out, is not a biologist. Nor is he a historian or an ambassador. He's a former salesman who gives speeches to civic and social groups. Only the person who invites him to speak knows that he offers more than a dozen phony expert speeches on all sorts of topics. William's speech lasts until he's found out or runs out of material from his hastily created notes. Then he continues with stories about his experiences as a real person and as a would-be expert. "The joy of this job is that I'm always thinking on my feet," he says. "I never know how it will go, because no two experiences are the same."

People over age fifty who said they defined their lives around multiple roles were 20 percent more likely to be highly satisfied.

Grocer 2001

80

Put Stuff in Its Place

Understand the limited value of the things you can buy. The pursuit of whatever is bigger and newer traps people in an endless, and unfulfilling, cycle of getting and spending money. Define the things you truly value, and do not let yourself get caught buying for the sake of buying.

Pam helps people organize their stuff. "People get too much stuff, and it starts to take over their homes," she says. Pam changes the layout of closets, helps consolidate things, and ultimately tries to get owners to consider how much of what they have is really necessary. "Then after I'm done, if I've done a good job, their home functions better and stuff won't overwhelm them," she adds.

Her theory is that clutter drains energy and creativity, and that getting rid of it opens the door to greater productivity, personal growth, and peace.

It was a sad irony for Pam when her aunt died and Pam inherited her home. "It was packed with things in no discernible order.

There were valuable items mixed in with things that were sentimentally valuable mixed in with things that seemed to have no purpose whatsoever," she recalls.

Pam encourages people to think through what they have and what they value, especially items of personal and family significance. "People think they will have endless time to sort through things and make sense of it all," she says. "But it slips down on the list, and if they don't act, many unique and personally treasured items get lost in the crowd."

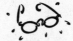

Among participants in one study, those whose values were the most materialistic rated their lives as the least satisfying.

Ryan and Dziurawiec 2001

81

Seek Meaning

You want to live in a nice home and enjoy certain luxuries. You want to have a certain position of respect in your community. But no accomplishment will be of value to you unless there is meaning in your life. Unless you know what you are living for, the style in which you are living will not matter one bit. Seek the meaning in your life and in what you do, and you will feel satisfaction in the process, regardless of the outcome.

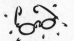

Professor Joe Talbot runs a research center on aging. He deals with quality-of-life issues for people in their fifties, sixties, and beyond. Professor Talbot says the question of meaning in life takes on a special significance when people reach their fifties.

"Before age fifty," he explains, "most people have almost an automatic identity either through their work or through their family or both. There is little need or time for big questions of meaning, because the influences of life are so powerful and ever present. You do what you have to do, and you rarely ask why.

"But then you reach a stage in life when you enter a new phase. You may be winding down a career, you may be retiring, your children may be off raising children of their own. And for the first time, you are confronted with a combination of big questions and big openings. Because now you can go in a new direction. You can redefine yourself, because the responsibilities you have carried are no longer there."

Professor Talbot says the greatest gift people can give themselves is the opportunity to think through what they really believe and value. "We accept so much automatically. The beauty of finding a meaning and purpose in our lives is that it is totally our own creation," he says.

Professor Talbot calls it a process of finding "our voices." He says there is reason for optimism because "many people succeed in making new meaning. Their lives make sense to them. They're able to wake up in the morning with a sense of giftedness. They find tasks and projects, commitments and ties that make sense of their days."

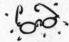

Those with a modest income who felt there was meaning in their lives were twice as likely to experience life satisfaction as were those who were wealthier but who felt that their lives lacked a sense of meaning.

Debats 1999

82

We Never Outgrow Jealousy

Some behaviors that we regard as silly we will eventually outgrow. Others we will never rid ourselves of. Jealousy is one of the latter. We make constant comparisons between ourselves and others, and we keep constant watch over the possibility that someone might intrude into our relationships. Understand this instinct in yourself and in others, and acknowledge that, even with the wisdom of years, you need to actively control your inclination to be jealous.

The radio host Diane Rehm's distinctive voice is known to the millions who listen to her talk show. For more than four decades, she has been married to attorney John Rehm.

People married for that long are expected to be experts in having a happy relationship. Yet John and Diane say that's hardly the case. "We have struggled mightily," John says, cautioning that "thinking everything can be perfect" is one of the most formidable challenges that couples face.

Though they have remained faithful to each other, friendships sometimes became sources of suspicion. At one point, John briefly moved out.

But jealousies have raged in many directions. When they were first married, Diane felt that John paid more attention to his mother's priorities than to hers. "I felt I was a second-class citizen in my own family," Diane says.

Meanwhile, John's professional life was coming to an end as Diane's continued to expand. John admits to thinking less and less of his own accomplishments as Diane's success grew. When someone referred to John as "Mr. Diane Rehm," those feelings only intensified.

Both John and Diane recognized that such jealousies have been a part of their lives, and they both have resolved not to take them out on each other. "The bad feelings come. The question is what you do with them. We recognize them, but we realize there is something more important to our love than our feelings of jealousy," John says.

Even among those happily married for more than two decades, a majority have concerns about the possibility that their spouse may commit adultery.

Shackelford and Buss 2000

83

Cherish Your Heritage

Where you and your ancestors came from tells you a lot about yourself, about your past, and even about your future. Whether you are keeping family stories alive, continuing traditions, or just appreciating your background, you benefit from staying in touch with the history of those whom you consider to be your people, because it gives you a sense of belonging in an often isolating world.

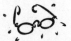

Nearing fifty, Vince is one of the youngest members of his Chicago-area Italian-American club. He appreciates the culture, the cuisine, and the traditions of his heritage, and he enjoys sharing them across the generations.

The city's Italian-American festival "was so much a part of our summer when we were growing up," says Vince. "My parents made it important to me, and I want to share that with other people."

But he's concerned that older club members have not done a very good job of making their organization relevant to the next generation. "Younger people in here, it's like they're the hired help.

They tell them, 'Here, just set up these chairs,'" Vince says. "What a shame it would be for people to lose touch with their history, with this community. I want to see us do a better job of sharing the celebration of our heritage with people of all ages."

Vince is trying hard to see that long-standing traditions continue, and maybe even improve. He has worked on changing the route of the city's Columbus Day parade so that it reaches more of the Italian-Americans across the city.

The good news for Vince is that he's "seeing a lot of interest in learning about Italian culture in different ways. And that makes you feel like you have a good connection to people."

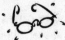

People who were interested in their family and ethnic histories were 6 percent more likely to feel satisfied with their lives.

Mowrer and McCarver 2002

84

Share Your Fun

The regular leisure activities of our lives—watching our favorite television show, listening to music, engaging in a hobby, playing a game—are a great source of comfort, amusement, and pleasure. But their value is much greater if we share them. Comedies become funnier, music more moving, hobbies more interesting, and games more compelling. More important, the social connections we build in this way will retain their importance long after we lose interest in the original activity.

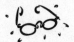

In her spare time, Kemvia had been known to drive race cars around a track at top speeds. It was thrilling, exciting, and a bit scary.

Today, when she isn't planning excursions, she spends a lot of her time behind the wheel working as a parks-and-recreation supervisor, escorting groups of senior citizens on trips across the state of Virginia. They visit all kinds of parks and natural wonders, and different cities and towns throughout the state.

"The excitement of these adventures gets your blood flowing, and that's why we do different things," Kemvia says. "We go with about twenty-five people. Folks come out with their friends and see things and places they've never seen before."

"I just love Kemvia, and I love these trips. She's a real good travel guide, and we all have such fun together," says one of her regular participants.

And the excitement of driving is there for Kemvia, too. "It's wicked out there on the road," she says. "Someone will cut the bus off, and then my passengers will raise Cain in the back at other drivers. And I say, 'You tell 'em.'" Her job and her hobby finally came together when she took the seniors on a tour of a racetrack.

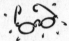

People who said they frequently engaged in leisure activities with others were 31 percent more likely to typically be in a good mood than people who engaged in such activities by themselves.

Hills and Argyle 1998

85

Pay Attention to Your Dreams

Your dreams are more than a fleeting source of nighttime entertainment. Much like the dashboard of your car, which tells you
what's going on under the hood, your dreams tell you what's going
on inside your system. Pay attention to what's happening in your
dreams, remember them, and write them down, because they are
an important clue to what you are really feeling.

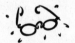

Right after finishing school, Monica started working as a flight
attendant. She began with short flights—"milk runs"—back and
forth between nearby cities. Over time she moved on to international flights and had her pick of European and South American
destinations.

She enjoyed the work. She enjoyed the schedule, which allowed
her to work for a series of days and then take a series of days off.
And she loved the opportunity to see the world. "For me, the job
was everything I could have wanted," she recalls.

Monica had plans of staying in the air until she retired. But then
the work started to wear on her physically and mentally. "When I

hit fifty," Monica says, "it really began to be physically draining. Then I started to feel less enthusiastic for everything. It became harder to laugh off irritating things that hadn't bothered me before—like the tug of war with a passenger who says, 'I won't put that under my seat.' I just didn't want to deal with certain trivialities anymore."

But Monica really decided she had to make a change only when she started having a series of dreams in which she felt continually isolated and scared. "There was so much negativity in my days that even when I was asleep, my brain was focused on negative things," Monica says. "It was as if my body was sending me a message that it was determined I get, one way or the other."

Six months later she was working in sales. With her new job firmly on solid ground, her dreams returned to much less turbulent subjects.

People who regularly dream about negative or traumatic events are 13 percent less likely to feel satisfied with their lives.

Kroth et al. 2002

86

All the Time Is Too Much

Time with loved ones and friends is wonderful. But spending all your time with a loved one or friend will be counterproductive. Neither of you will enjoy the time as much, nerves will fray, and instead of feeling better for the time invested, you will both feel worse. Spend time together, but not all the time.

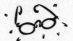

Adam and Kay have been married for more than forty years. They have three children and seven grandchildren. They consider themselves blessed, and they treasure the time they spend together as a couple and as a family.

But they realize that part of what makes that time special is that they live their own lives, too.

Adam and Kay have kept a routine they had when they both worked. Now, instead of going out the door to work and then returning each night to have dinner together, Adam and Kay separately plan their day's activities until dinnertime, when they eat together and spend the evening together.

"Two people sitting around all day get under each other's feet. Little things start to irritate you, and then everybody's grumpy," Kay says. "Instead, he has a day. I have a day. And we can look forward to being together for supper and talking about our days."

They approach time with their family the same way. "When we visit, we make it clear that everybody should keep on living their lives," Kay explains. "Twenty-four hours a day of grandma and grandpa is not what any eight-year-old wants. But when we all take a walk together after dinner, it's the greatest feeling of togetherness you could hope for."

Maximizing leisure time spent together reduced marital satisfaction by 30 percent among those married for more than three decades.

Crawford et al. 2002

87

Regrets Hold Us Back

We can't change the past; we can't improve it. Dwelling on past disappointments can change the future, but only to make it worse. Relieve yourself of the burden of past regrets. Your goal is to set the best course for the future, not to suffer over the imperfections of the past.

On the surface, Nathan would seem to be a good candidate for living with a heavy load of regret. He put every penny he had, and even some that he borrowed, into starting a business that never prospered. He came home from work one day and found that his wife of twelve years had packed up her things and left him. "Didn't even say good-bye," he says. And three years later, his home was flooded in a hurricane.

"You know what I regret?" Nathan asks. "Nothing.

"I don't pretend I didn't make mistakes. I made a lot. And it's clear I had some poor runs of luck. But the way I look at it, it's the good and the bad that made me who I am. If you go back and change something, who knows what you are left with?

"And thinking about what I've lost gets in the way of thinking about what I have—which is a long time in front of me to do things right or to do things better. I can't let regret stop me now. Then it would be all over."

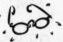

Those who frequently thought about mistakes that they had made and regrets that they had were 17 percent less likely to feel happy with their lives.

Jokisaari 2003

174

88

See Your Goals

When we become adults and start careers or families, we have numerous goals for our lives. We can see them clearly and know what we have to do to move toward them. Yet the same should be true at any stage of life. Goals give us focus and purpose. Regardless of what is important to you now, your goals should be clear and visible every day.

With his camera always at the ready, Bob Jordan has photographed hurricanes, governors, presidents, a war, and championship basketball games. In more than three decades as a newspaper photographer, he's handled assignments of every imaginable kind.

Bob says that the key to his career in newspapers, which he began as an apprentice, helping to print the paper, has been a constant dedication to the goal of doing his job as well as he can do it.

"I had this noble vision of putting something together that people were going to read a few hours later," Bob says. "Even though I was walking in at the lowest level, I felt a tremendous responsibility to do it right." Bob took seriously his father's belief that nothing in work is guaranteed but that "the one thing you can control is how hard you work."

Bob's career in the printing room advanced gradually until he decided to seek a photographer's position. It was a chance for him to take the pictures he'd been hard at work printing in the paper.

Bob had no degree in photojournalism, no experience, not even a basic understanding of the tools of the job. "But I had the goal to do the job well," Bob recalls. "And for me, it was a dream come true." He studied the techniques of the more experienced colleagues he would meet at events, and he soaked up all the information he could.

Today Bob is valued as a mentor to countless photojournalists. And even with all the experience he has, he still gets to events in advance of his media colleagues so that he can be better prepared. And though he's a skilled veteran in the trade, he still gets nervous before every assignment. "I've never lost that, " Bob says, "whether it's going out and shooting a head shot or covering a basketball game. Your name goes on the picture. I want it to be the best it can be.

"Some people might try to coast as they get older. But that's not for me. I don't see why, as you get older, you can't get better."

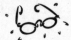

People who could identify a goal they were pursuing were 19 percent more likely to feel satisfied with their lives and 26 percent more likely to feel positive about themselves.

Krueger 1998

89

Give the Gift of Yourself

Giving gifts to loved ones, especially children, can be a challenge. The stores are stuffed with increasingly expensive items that we hope will function and hope will be of some value to the recipient. But the chase for the better gift is ultimately fruitless. Little enduring satisfaction comes to the giver or to the recipient, and the nature of the gift is often soon forgotten. Instead of busting your bank account for the next round of gifts, give something of yourself. Though some of us have the talent to actually make gifts, anyone can make special plans to spend time with a loved one—a gift that will hold lasting meaning.

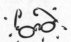

Surveying the living room after the birthday party for her seven-year-old grandson, Bobby, was over, Claire felt overwhelmed by all the boxes and scraps of wrapping paper—but even more so by the piles of toys. "I thought, 'He's only one boy. How could he possibly play with all those things? He'd need to be up twenty-four hours a day just to get to some of them,'" she says.

Although Clair loves her grandson and loves for him to have gifts, she asked herself if there wasn't a better way. "I know he likes Spider-Man. I went to the store and found out that you can't just give him Spider-Man, because now there's 212 different Spider-Men—different costumes, different poses, and so forth. Well, how many Spider-Men does one boy need?"

She talked it over with her daughter and son-in-law, and they agreed that the toys had gotten out of control. And so for Bobby's next birthday, Claire decided to try something else.

Her gift, she decided, would be a day trip to wherever Bobby wanted to go within fifty miles. "I wrapped up a map, with a circle drawn fifty miles around his home," she explains. Then the two of them talked about all the different places they could go. "It was so much different than just throwing another toy on the pile," she says. "Here we were, planning this together, talking, and then there was the day itself."

Ultimately they decided on a trip to a park that offers public tours of a cave. Having never been in a cave, Claire was a bit anxious about the visit. But afterward she thought she had never given a better gift. "I think Bobby enjoyed it," she says, "and I know I'll never forget it."

Among parents studied, greater expenditures for family gifts actually reduced satisfaction with family holidays by 2 percent.

Kasser and Sheldon 2002

90

Boredom Is the Enemy

There is only one true waste of time: boredom. Boredom is the feeling that there is nothing worth doing. Your time becomes a hurdle to be overcome instead of a resource to be treasured. Doing absolutely anything is more productive than boredom.

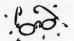

"What's the expression about how something boring is about as exciting as watching paint dry?" Harold asks. "Well, I'll tell you, there were days I would have signed on for that in a minute. 'Which wall will be dry first?' I'd wonder. 'It looks dry on top, but I bet you can't touch it yet.'"

Harold took early retirement from a career in the construction industry with the idea that he could do all the things he'd always wanted to do but never had the time for. "But then after I did all the things I'd always wanted to do, I was lost," he recalls.

Harold looked at the lives of his retired friends and found that although no two were doing the same thing, they all seemed to be doing something: "Some 'un-retired' themselves. Some threw themselves into volunteering. Some had big family responsibilities like helping to care for grandchildren. They just didn't seem to be making a life out of nothing, which is what I was trying to do."

Harold didn't really want a job, but when a friend suggested there were other ways he could put his knowledge and background to use, he headed to his local planning and zoning committee. The committee advises the city council on proposed new construction projects, judging whether they are appropriate for the town and whether the plans fit the character of the neighborhood involved. Harold was appointed to a seat on the committee and found himself fascinated by the task. "You really see the town on another level from this vantage point—and it always gives me something to think about," he says.

People over fifty who frequently experienced feelings of boredom were three times more likely to describe their lives as empty and two times more likely to be apathetic about the future.

Bargdill 2000

91

Redefine Career

At one time, a career for most people meant a multidecade commitment to a single employer. As the economy changed, many adapted to the expectation that a career might involve not only many employers but a number of different specialties. Your task now is to adapt to the meaning of career again. Whether or not you will be working for pay, you can have a career. And you can have it on your terms, for your purposes. Your career is whatever you think is the most valuable pursuit in your life.

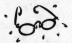

At various times, Howard ran an insurance company and owned racehorses. When he was in his late thirties, his doctors advised him to stop working, warning that otherwise his fragile health would worsen. He did stop working for a while. But, dabbling in a few tasks here and there, he found his early retirement to be unsatisfying.

In his mid-fifties, though, Howard found an opportunity that inspired him. He decided to take his career in another direction as he formed a small company that purchases prescription medicine in Canada and imports it to the United States.

The practice remains legally questionable. The federal government does not allow prescription drugs to be imported, but several local governments are actively buying medicine from Howard and his competitors.

Part traveling salesman, part social activist, Howard spends countless hours in rental cars and hotel rooms, traveling around the United States to meet with senior citizens and local government officials. He tells them that they are being overcharged by the drug companies. "The United States of America pays a ridiculous price, and the seniors carry the burden, and it's wrong," Howard tells his listeners.

Howard does not know how long this work will be possible. "If the laws change to make this easier or harder, either way I'm out of business," he says. But he does know he's enjoyed the work. And, he adds, "I'm back. This might end, but I will find something else that needs my attention."

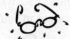

People over sixty who were the most flexible in defining the concept of a career were 36 percent less likely to feel disappointed with retirement.

Crosnoe and Elder 2002

92

Travel the Stable Road

Peaks give way to valleys. It is a simple law of nature. Your emotional highs will give way to emotional lows. The best route to consistently feeling good is to value the plateau.

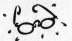

The first baseman had cancer. The second baseman, shortstop, and third baseman have all had heart attacks. "And if you think that's bad, wait until you hear about the shape of our outfielders," says Ted.

On this softball team for men in their fifties, sixties, and seventies, major health difficulties have been a part of almost every player's life.

And yet, those problems are rarely discussed. "We don't talk medicine," Ted says. "Very seldom do we talk about ailments and hurts, because we've all had them. So we play through them and don't think about it. We're having fun."

They make an exception for on-field injuries. Ted and his teammates love to talk, for example, about the time he tripped while rounding third base and broke his leg. When it happened, the first words he heard from a league official were not "Are you OK?" or "Do you need some help?" Instead, says Ted, "The guy says to me, 'You're out.'"

The bottom line for Ted and his teammates is simple. Ted puts it this way: "We can all still hit. And the rest of the day goes a little smoother after you've knocked one over the right fielder's head."

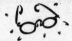

People who experienced fewer dramatic changes in mood were 21 percent more likely to maintain an optimistic outlook on life.

Hills and Argyle 2001

93

It's Less What Happened
Than What Happened Next

You will face difficult times. Everyone does. But how things turn out for you has less to do with the events themselves than with your response to them. Answer the challenges that are presented to you, persevere through the traumas that may occur, and you will be made stronger for your life ahead.

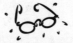

Doug had lost his wife to illness only a year before. Grief was still fresh within him. When there was a knock on his door early one morning, his first thought was that whatever would bring someone to his home at that hour could not be good.

Soon he would learn that his brother, one of the people he was closest to, had been killed by what the media called "the sniper," which turned out to be two serial killers who had been terrorizing the Washington, D.C., area in 2002.

Doug had seen footage on the news about the string of deadly crimes and had discussed it with his brother. But he didn't imagine for a moment when he had heard the latest tragic report that the unnamed victim was his brother.

When his wife died, Doug figured that he could take one of two paths: he could be bitter and angry at the cruel loss, or he could accept that she was in a better place and that he would have to go on living his life. He tried to hold those same thoughts as he faced the excruciating task of telling his elderly parents that their son was gone.

It was more painful than he could describe. But as a family, Doug, his parents, and his other relatives resolved to not let the pain destroy them. "We decided that we had to be strong enough not to question or become bitter," he says. "It's not easy, but we still need to realize all the wonderful things we've been privileged to experience.

"A family is like a table, with each person a leg. We feel the loss, and it aches. But we're going to have to fight through this and live with a wobbly table."

The length of time that personal tragedies continued to affect life satisfaction ranged from days to decades, depending on the person's response to the stressors.

Hamarat et al. 2001

94

You Define Success

It is all up to you. No outcome can force you to feel successful—or to feel that you failed. No other person can convince you that what you have is good or bad. It is up to you to define what life means and where you stand. Define your life for yourself.

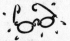

Vola didn't travel the usual path to her career or in her career.

She started in public service in a sense: on the sidewalk outside city hall. She participated in various protests, seeking fair treatment for the citizens of Alexandria, Virginia, just across the river from Washington, D.C. Later she took a low-level job in city hall.

When the city conducted a national search to hire a city manager, the top professional job in the city government, they decided that the best person for the job already worked for them. When Vola was named city manager, she became only the third woman in the country to run a city of more than one hundred thousand.

City managers usually don't last very long in their jobs. They must constantly maintain the support of the mayor and city council members, and many who succeed in their work soon seek larger cities to run.

In her fifteen years on the job, though, Vola has held the support of four different mayors and dozens of city council members. And she never sought a position in a bigger city.

"I love what I do," she says. "I think that some managers plan to build their careers moving along, almost as if you were in the military moving around. But I lived in Alexandria before taking this job, and I'm going to live in Alexandria after this job. I think I know the city, and I've been very fortunate to work with terrific mayors and city councils.

"It's how you define success. There are a lot of nomads out there who decide they want to keep moving to a bigger city. But being city manager in Alexandria was, in my mind, a success."

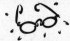

Personal feelings of fulfillment are four times better at predicting life satisfaction than are any objective or structured measures of life outcomes.

Scannell, Allen, and Burton 2002

95

Never Stop Learning

There is really only one way things ever improve. Progress comes from learning. The learning may come from a teacher, from a book, or from experience and personal curiosity. But no matter what its origin, learning is the essence not only of a society's progress, but of personal progress. The decision and commitment to continue learning are the decision and commitment to continue truly living—and to live not just as you always have but as you truly can.

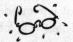

Charlotte retired from a career in retail sales. She moved to Florida with her husband, but she found that no combination of golf, shuffleboard, and bingo could hold her attention.

Then she wandered over to the local college.

She found not only that she was eligible to audit traditional courses but that the school had an entire program geared just for seniors: classes with no homework or tests but plenty of lectures and discussions. "And these weren't frivolous topics—serious things like foreign policy and advances in biomedicine," Charlotte explains.

She enrolled in a course and loved it. "I was looking around for something to fill a void, and I found it," says Charlotte. "It used to be, at sixty-five, you went out to pasture. But the senior community has found out that the brain is a muscle and that unless you use it, it atrophies."

Charlotte has been inspired not just by the faculty but by her fellow students. "No one has to push them, shove them, or beat them over the head to be here. They're here by choice. And they take this opportunity very seriously," says Charlotte. "My fellow students are always challenging the instructor with interesting questions, and they won't let anyone get away with superficial answers. More than anything, these students bring the experience of a working life with them.

"And the best part is, after every class I go home thinking."

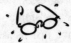

People over the age of fifty who said they continued to learn about topics that interested them were 18 percent more likely to feel satisfied with their lives and 43 percent more likely to feel vital.

Helterbran 1999

96

View Your Life as a Choice

In some sense, everything that has ever happened to you reflects the collective result of an almost infinite series of choices. From the trivial to the crucial, your choices brought you to this moment. In recognizing that your choices matter and that they guide you, you are taking on a burden, but you are also giving yourself the opportunity to accept life's outcomes and to decide what kind of future you want.

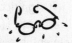

Part of the year it was much too cold. And part of the year it was much too hot. But before he retired Tom treated each day delivering the mail in the same Indianapolis neighborhood as a chance to do work he enjoyed, surrounded by people he liked.

Tom made friends with the residents as he delivered the pieces of paper that defined their lives: wedding announcements, college acceptances, job offers, love letters. He went to their parties and their funerals. He cherished his job for its simplicity, the friendliness of those he delivered to, and the routine and rhythms of his days.

Over the course of his career, Tom had many opportunities to switch to a different route. He could have had one that involved less walking or less climbing. But he always declined, because he didn't want to leave the neighborhood he felt so close to.

"I felt very comfortable being out here, seeing the same people all the time. I've made friends with them," Tom says. "A lot of the people have gone through pretty much every stage of my life as it developed over the years."

Walking up and down the streets, Tom served as the collective eyes and ears of the neighborhood. One time Tom foiled a home robbery when he saw two men inside a house and knew that the owner was away and that no one should have been in there.

Tom's co-workers have long admired his attitude. "He said, 'This is the work I chose.' He never complained," one says. "He loved getting up at the crack of dawn, because he was going to get out there and he was appreciated."

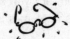

People who said they felt significant disappointment with the outcome of their lives were 14 percent less likely to dwell on that disappointment if they viewed their lives' outcome as a reflection of their choices and not as something they were powerless over.

Robinson-Rowe 2002

97

Make Your Mark on the Next Generation

We need to know that we have accomplished something. We need to know that what we have done has had some lasting value. There is no better way to meet those goals than to influence the next generation. Whether it is through family, a friendship, a community group, or even through benefiting people we'll never know, we need to see that what we've done continues. Keep the next generation in the forefront of your goals, and rest assured that their futures will benefit.

Rita didn't have a lot. She didn't have a lot of money, and she didn't have a lot of free time.

But the time Rita did have she loved to spend in her garden. Rita planted almost every inch of her backyard with vegetables. Every day her neighbors would see her out there in her boots before and after work, weeding, planting, watering, and caring for her tomatoes, corn, squash, carrots, and cucumbers.

But it's what she did with her vegetables that her neighbors were most impressed by. Living in a poverty-stricken area, Rita not only was willing to share what she had but insisted that her neighbors share in the bounty.

And for those who had no idea what to do with a squash, Rita was ready with recipes and ideas.

Health problems eventually slowed Rita down and kept her from her garden. Instead of missing the season, though, her neighbors pitched in and planted it for her.

"I swear, the only reason half the children in the neighborhood ever saw a fresh vegetable was because of Rita," one neighbor says. "You don't meet too many inspirational people, but Rita is an inspiration."

Age, income, and health are four times less likely to predict whether a person is happy than is whether the person feels he or she is having a positive effect on a younger person.

Azarow 2003

98

Why Not Be Optimistic?

Without hope, what would you ever have tried? Nothing you've accomplished, nothing you've enjoyed would have been possible unless you had first seen possibilities. Seize that view to guide you to the future you desire.

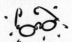

Just starting out in the business world, Charles Blasband wanted a job working for a dynamic employer, where he had the potential to advance.

Charles got a call from the head of the Citrus County, Florida, hospital inviting him to interview for a job as the hospital's chief financial officer.

When he drove to the hospital, he thought he must have gotten the address wrong. He was staring at an unassuming one-story building that hardly resembled any hospital he'd ever seen when he was growing up in Philadelphia.

After a tour of the facility, the hospital's CEO took Charles out for a drive in the surrounding area. Charles thought he was wasting his time.

Driving through rural farmland, the CEO told Charles that he thought the hospital had potential, that he thought Charles had potential, and that if he was as talented and dedicated as he appeared, Charles would be running the hospital before long.

Charles's skepticism melted away at the sound of the "magic words" that made him think there was something special in store for him at Citrus County Hospital. Sure enough, six years later Charles was promoted to CEO.

As the hospital grew, so, too, did Charles's responsibilities. Under his leadership the facility expanded its emergency room, added operating rooms, and erected a new building for physicians. He tripled the number of beds, and he created a heart-care facility offering the only open-heart procedures anywhere in the region.

The typical hospital executive stays on the job for about five years. More than twenty-five years later, Charles is still running Citrus County Hospital. "I first thought this was just a bump in the road," he says. "But then I thought it could be something more."

People with a tendency to see things optimistically were 42 percent less likely to feel burdened by their age and 29 percent more likely to feel a sense of well-being.

Lounsbury et al. 2003

99

There's No Deadline for Your Dreams

We spend our whole lives making plans. We set goals for ourselves in every part of our lives, and once in a while we look back and see what we've accomplished. Though it is reasonable to have a time frame for our lives and our goals, the truth is that the dreams we had when we were younger don't have an expiration date. Live your life toward your dreams. No one will ask you what day it is when you get there.

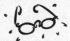

He has spent twenty years in the military. He's married and has six children. He drives a minivan.

And, he's playing college football for the University of South Carolina.

Tim Frisby went straight into the military after high school. He loved sports as a child and would have loved to go to college, but he felt that the military was his best career opportunity. Throughout his two decades of military service, he followed college football and his favorite team, South Carolina.

As an army ranger, he made fitness a constant part of his life, but he often thought of the day his military career would be over. "I dreamed of playing college football. It was in the back of my head every day," he recalls.

His teammates have nicknamed him "Pops." But although he's older than some of his teammates' parents, Tim spends not a moment wishing he was younger.

Tim's not out to prove a point, either. "I don't want to be a novelty," Tim says. "I don't want to be sitting on the sidelines, with people saying, 'That guy is thirty-nine, but he's not really contributing.' I want to contribute."

The South Carolina coaches rave about his attitude, his commitment, his work ethic, and his leadership abilities. "He sets an example for his teammates every day," one assistant coach says.

His military colleagues think he sets a shining example for them, too. "You're never too old to reach your goals," says one of his officers. "Tim's definitely a morale builder for these soldiers. They tend not to think about goals outside of the military, only within. But here is Tim, not only attaining his military goals but doing something remarkable outside the military."

People who felt they had reached their life dream were more likely to feel satisfied with their lives, but the age at which they reached that dream was unrelated to their level of satisfaction.

Krueger 1998

100

Do It Now

Nothing changes. Nothing matters. "You can't teach an old dog . . ." Well, you know the saying. These thoughts are the enemy of enjoying life. More important, they are not true. The most vital belief you need in order to live your life fully is that actions matter. Actions are called for. Actions are rewarded. Take action now. There's no reason you shouldn't, and many reasons you should.

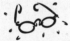

"I'm an action guy. I've got to be doing something," Dan says.

Dan spent a career fighting fires in upstate New York. He chose the work because he wanted to do something. "The fire department looked like it would be pretty exciting. Whenever I saw a fire truck race by with those guys hanging off the back, I said, 'That looks like something that would hold my attention,'" he recalls.

When Dan reached his mid-fifties, he had already surpassed the typical retirement age in his department. So he retired, at least in theory.

Before his papers were even complete, though, Dan found work with the Federal Emergency Management Agency.

"Retirement from the fire department hasn't made me slow down," he says. "It's an opportunity to speed up."

FEMA has sent him to Puerto Rico, Louisiana, Kentucky, New Jersey, New York City, and Iowa in the wake of floods, tornadoes, and other disasters, and Dan helps people put their lives back together.

"It's an exciting job," he says. "They call me and they say, 'Get your gear.' Then you get on the plane and go.

"In this job, you get to see parts of this country you don't normally see, and you don't do it as a tourist. You go to where something's happening. You help people. For a moment, you become part of the community." And, a few weeks later, "you do it again someplace else."

The feeling that any actions they took would be unlikely to produce results caused feelings of apathy and boredom in 74 percent of the participants in one study.

Bargdill 1998

Sources

Altus, D., and R. M. Mathews. 2000. "Examining Satisfaction of Older Home Owners with Intergenerational Homesharing." *Journal of Clinical Geropsychology* 6 (2): 139–47.

Amato, P., D. Johnson, A. Booth, and S. Rogers. 2003. "Continuity and Change in Marital Quality Between 1980 and 2000." *Journal of Marriage and Family* 65 (1): 1–22.

Auerbach, S., A. Penberthy, and D. Kiesler. 2004. "Opportunity for Control, Interpersonal Impacts, and Adjustment to a Long-Term Invasive Health Care Procedure." *Journal of Behavioral Medicine* 27 (1): 11–29.

Austrom, M., A. Perkins, T. Damush, and H. Hendrie. 2003. "Predictors of Life Satisfaction in Retired Physicians and Spouses." *Social Psychiatry and Psychiatric Epidemiology* 38 (3): 134–41.

Azarow, J. 2003. "Generativity and Well-Being: An Investigation of the Eriksonian Hypothesis." Ph.D. dissertation, Northwestern University.

Baerger, D., and D. McAdams. 1999. "Life Story Coherence and Its Relation to Psychological Well-Being." *Narrative Inquiry* 9 (1): 69–96.

Bargdill, R. 1998. "Being Bored with One's Life: An Empirical Phenomenological Study." Ph.D. dissertation, Duquesne University.

———. 2000. "The Study of Life Boredom." *Journal of Phenomenological Psychology* 31 (2): 188–219.

Berry, J., and E. Worthington. 2001. "Forgivingness, Relationship Quality, Stress While Imagining Relationship Events, and Physical and Mental Health." *Journal of Counseling Psychology* 48 (4): 447–55.

Bippus, A., and E. Rollin. 2003. "Attachment Style Differences in Relational Maintenance and Conflict Behaviors: Friends' Perceptions." *Communication Reports* 16 (2): 113–23.

Bozeman, D., P. Perrewe, W. Hochwarter, and R. Brymer. 2001. "Organizational Politics, Perceived Control, and Work Outcomes: Boundary Conditions on the Effects of Politics." *Journal of Applied Social Psychology* 31 (3): 486–503.

Burack, O., P. Jefferson, and L. Libow. 2002. "Individualized Music: A Route to Improving the Quality of Life for Long-Term Care Residents." *Activities, Adaptation and Aging* 27 (1): 63–76.

Cameron, P. 1972. "Stereotypes About Generational Fun and Happiness vs. Self-Appraised Fun and Happiness." *Gerontologist* 12 (2): 120–23.

Caughlin, J., and T. Golish. 2002. "An Analysis of the Association Between Topic Avoidance and Dissatisfaction: Comparing Perceptual and Interpersonal Explanations." *Communication Monographs* 69 (4): 275–95.

Chamberlain, J., and D. Haaga. 2001. "Unconditional Self-Acceptance and Psychological Health." *Journal of Rational-Emotive and Cognitive Behavior Therapy* 19 (3): 163–76.

Chen, C. 2001. "Aging and Life Satisfaction." *Social Indicators Research* 54 (1): 57–79.

Chen, Y., and B. King. 2002. "Intra- and Intergenerational Communication Satisfaction as a Function of an Individual's Age and Age Stereotypes." *International Journal of Behavioral Development* 26 (6): 562–70.

Christiansen, C. 2000. "Identity, Personal Projects and Happiness: Self Construction in Everyday Action." *Journal of Occupational Science* 7 (3): 98–107.

Clarke, S. 1998. "Taking Care: Women High School Teachers at Midlife and Midcareer." Ph.D. dissertation, University of Massachusetts.

Crawford, D., R. Houts, T. Huston, and L. George. 2002. "Compatibility, Leisure, and Satisfaction in Marital Relationships." *Journal of Marriage and Family* 64 (2): 433–49.

Crosnoe, R., and G. Elder. 2002. "Successful Adaptation in the Later Years: A Life Course Approach to Aging." *Social Psychology Quarterly* 65 (4): 309–28.

Debats, D. 1999. "Sources of Meaning: An Investigation of Significant Commitments in Life." *Journal of Humanistic Psychology* 39 (4): 30–57.

Di Bona, L. 2000. "What Are the Benefits of Leisure? An Exploration Using the Leisure Satisfaction Scale." *British Journal of Occupational Therapy* 63 (2): 50–58.

Diener, E., and M. Suh. 1998. "Subjective Well-Being and Age: An International Analysis." *Annual Review of Gerontology and Geriatrics* 17: 304–24

Donaghue, N., and B. Fallon. 2003. "Gender-Role Self-Stereotyping and the Relationship Between Equity and Satisfaction in Close Relationships." *Sex Roles* 48 (5–6): 217–30.

Dormann, C., and D. Zapf. 2001. "Job Satisfaction: A Meta-Analysis of Stabilities." *Journal of Organizational Behavior* 22 (5): 483–504.

Dube, L., M. Jodoin, and S. Kairouz. 1998. "On the Cognitive Basis of Subjective Well-Being Analysis: What Do Individuals Have to Say About It?" *Canadian Journal of Behavioural Science* 30 (1): 1–13.

Easterlin, R. 2001. "Life Cycle Welfare: Evidence and Conjecture." *Journal of Socio-Economics* 30 (1): 31–61.

Efklides, A., M. Kalaitzidou, and G. Chankin. 2003. "Subjective Quality of Life in Old Age in Greece: The Effect of Demographic Factors, Emotional State and Adaptation to Aging." *European Psychologist* 8 (3): 178–91.

Field, D. 1981. "Retrospective Reports by Healthy Intelligent Elderly People of Personal Events of Their Adult Lives." *International Journal of Behavioral Development* 4 (1): 77–97.

Finkenauer, C., and H. Hazam. 2000. "Disclosure and Secrecy in Marriage: Do Both Contribute to Marital Satisfaction?" *Journal of Social and Personal Relationships* 17 (2): 245–63.

Fouquereau, E., A. Fernandez, and E. Mullet. 2001. "Evaluation of Determinants of Retirement Satisfaction Among Workers and Retired People." *Social Behavior and Personality* 29 (8): 777–86.

Francis, L., and J. Bolger. 1997. "Personality and Psychological Well-Being in Later Life." *Irish Journal of Psychology* 18 (4): 444–47.

Francis, L., S. Jones, and C. Wilcox. 2000. "Religiosity and Happiness: During Adolescence, Young Adulthood, and Later Life." *Journal of Psychology and Christianity* 19 (3): 245–57.

Freeman, L. D. Templer, and C. Hill. 1999. "The Relationship Between Adult Happiness and Self-Appraised Childhood Happiness and Events." *Journal of Genetic Psychology* 160 (1): 46–54.

Frey, B., and A. Stutzer. 2000. "Happiness Prospers in Democracy." *Journal of Happiness Studies* 1 (3): 79–102.

Frijters, P. 2000. "Do Individuals Try to Maximize General Satisfaction?" *Journal of Economic Psychology* 21 (3): 281–304.

Gerdtham, U., and M. Johannesson. 2001. "The Relationship Between Happiness, Health, and Social Economic Factors." *Journal of Socio-Economics* 30 (6): 553–57.

Glenn, N. 1975. "Psychological Well-Being in the Postparental Stage: Some Evidence from National Surveys." *Journal of Marriage and the Family* 37 (1): 105–10.

Gotlib, I., E. Krasnoperova, D. Neubauer Yue, and J. Joormann. 2004. "Attentional Biases for Negative Interpersonal Stimuli in Clinical Depression." *Journal of Abnormal Psychology* 113 (1): 121–35.

Grocer, S. 2001. "Life Satisfaction and Well-Being for College-Educated, Midlife, African American Women." Ph.D. dissertation, Howard University.

Gross, N., and S. Simmons. 2002. "Intimacy as a Double-Edged Phenomenon? An Empirical Test of Giddens." *Social Forces* 81 (2): 531–55.

Grossbaum, M., and G. Bates. 2002. "Correlates of Psychological Well-Being at Midlife: The Role of Generativity, Agency and Communion, and Narrative Themes." *International Journal of Behavioral Development* 26 (2): 120–27.

Halford, W. K., E. Keefer, and S. Osgarby. 2002. "'How Has the Week Been for You Two?' Relationship Satisfaction and Hindsight Memory Biases in Couples' Reports of Relationship Events." *Cognitive Therapy and Research* 26 (6): 759–73.

Hamarat, E., D. Thompson, K. Zabrucky, and D. Steele. 2001. "Perceived Stress and Coping Resource Availability as Predictors of Life Satisfaction in Young, Middle-Aged, and Older Adults." *Experimental Aging Research* 27 (2): 181–96.

Hart, P. 1999. "Predicting Employee Life Satisfaction: A Coherent Model of Personality, Work, and Nonwork Experiences, and Domain Satisfactions." *Journal of Applied Psychology* 84 (4): 564–84.

Helterbran, V. 1999. "Lifelong Learning: A Qualitative Study of Adult Self-Direction, Motivation to Learn, and Self-Efficacy in a Learning Society." Ph.D. dissertation, Duquesne University.

Hershey, D., J. Jacobs-Lawson, and K. Neukam. 2002. "Influences of Age and Gender on Workers' Goals for Retirement." *International Journal of Aging and Human Development* 55 (2): 163–79.

Hildreth, G., P. Dilworth-Anderson, and S. Rabe. 1983. "Family and School Life of Women over Age Fifty Who Are in College." *Educational Gerontology* 9 (4): 339–50.

Hills, P., and M. Argyle. 1998. "Positive Moods Derived from Leisure and Their Relationship to Happiness and Personality." *Personality and Individual Differences* 25 (3): 523–35.

———. 2001. "Emotional Stability as a Major Dimension of Happiness." *Personality and Individual Differences* 31 (8): 1357–64.

Hochwarter, W., G. Ferris, P. Perrewe, L. Witt, and C. Kiewitz. 2001. "A Note on the Nonlinearity of the Age-Job-Satisfaction Relationship." *Journal of Applied Social Psychology* 31 (6): 1223–37.

Hsieh, C. 2000. "Trends in Financial Satisfaction Among Middle-Age and Old-Age Americans, 1972–1996." *International Journal of Aging and Human Development* 51 (2): 105–13.

Hurd, L. 1999. "'We're Not Old!': Older Women's Negotiation of Aging and Oldness." *Journal of Aging Studies* 13 (4): 419–39.

Ikeuchi, H., and T. Fujihara. 2000. "The Effects of Loss of Material Possessions and Social Support Network on the Quality of Life." *Japanese Journal of Social Psychology* 16 (2): 92–102.

Isaacowitz, D., G. Vaillant, and M. Seligman. 2003. "Strengths and Satisfaction Across the Adult Lifespan." *International Journal of Aging and Human Development* 57 (2): 181–201.

Jokisaari, M. 2003. "Regret Appraisals, Age, and Subjective Well-Being." *Journal of Research in Personality* 37 (6): 487–503.

Kasser, T., and K. Sheldon. 2002. "What Makes for a Merry Christmas?" *Journal of Happiness Studies* 3 (4): 313–29.

Kaye, L., L. Alexander, and S. Kauffman. 1999. "Factors Contributing to Job Quality and Satisfaction Among Ethnically Diverse, Lower Income, Elderly Part-Timers." *Journal of Gerontological Social Work* 31 (1–2): 143–66.

Keyes, C. 2000. "Subjective Change and Its Consequences for Emotional Well-Being." *Motivation and Emotion* 24 (2): 67–84.

Kim, I., and C. Kim. 2003. "Patterns of Family Support and the Quality of Life of the Elderly." *Social Indicators Research* 62 (1–3): 437–54.

King, L., and C. Napa. 1998. "What Makes a Life Good?" *Journal of Personality and Social Psychology* 75 (1): 156–65.

Kinnier, R., N. Tribbensee, C. Rose, and S. Vaughan. 2001. "In the Final Analysis: More Wisdom from People Who Have Faced Death." *Journal of Counseling and Development* 79 (2): 171–77.

Kroth, J., A. Daline, D. Longstreet, M. Nelson, and L. O'Neal. 2002. "Sleep, Dreams, and Job Satisfaction." *Psychological Reports* 90 (3): 876–78.

Krueger, R. 1998. "The Status of Perceived Dream Fulfillment in Midlife Males." Ph.D. dissertation, California School of Professional Psychology.

Larsen, J., A. P. McGraw, and J. Cacioppo. 2001. "Can People Feel Happy and Sad at the Same Time?" *Journal of Personality and Social Psychology* 81 (4): 684–96.

Lavee, Y., and R. Katz. 2002. "Division of Labor, Perceived Fairness, and Marital Quality." *Journal of Marriage and Family* 64 (1): 27–39.

Lennings, C. 2000. "Optimism, Satisfaction and Time Perspective in the Elderly." *International Journal of Aging and Human Development* 51 (3): 167–81.

Logan, J., R. Ward, and G. Spitze. 1992. "As Old As You Feel: Age Identity in Middle and Later Life." *Social Forces* 71 (2) : 451–67.

Lounsbury, J., J. Loveland, E. Sundstrom, and L. Gibson. 2003. "An Investigation of Personality Traits in Relation to Career Satisfaction." *Journal of Career Assessment* 11 (3): 287–307.

Lu, L., and J. Bin Shih. 1997. "Sources of Happiness: A Qualitative Approach." *Journal of Social Psychology* 137 (2): 181–88.

Lucas, J., and R. Heady. 2002. "Flextime Commuters and Their Driver Stress, Feelings of Time Urgency, and Commute Satisfaction." *Journal of Business and Psychology* 16 (4): 565–72.

Mather, M., and L. Carstensen. 2003. "Aging and Attentional Biases for Emotional Faces." *Psychological Science* 14 (5): 409–15.

McAllister, D., and G. Bigley. 2002. "Work Context and the Definition of Self: How Organizational Care Influences Organization-Based Self-Esteem." *Academy of Management Journal* 45 (5): 894–904.

McAuley, E., B. Blissmer, D. Marquez, and G. Jerome. 2000. "Social Relations, Physical Activity and Well-Being in Older Adults." *Preventive Medicine* 31 (5): 608–17.

McGuinn, K., and P. Mosher-Ashley. 2000. "Participation in Recreational Activities and Its Effect on Perception of Life Satisfaction in Residential Settings." *Activities, Adaptation and Aging* 25 (1): 77–86.

Meeks, S., and S. Murrell. 2001. "Contribution of Education to Health and Life Satisfaction in Older Adults Mediated by Negative Affect." *Journal of Aging and Health* 13 (1): 92–119.

Mehlsen, M., M. Platz, and P. Fromholt. 2003. "Life Satisfaction Across the Life Course: Evaluations of the Most and Least Satisfying Decades of Life." *International Journal of Aging and Human Development* 57 (3): 217–36.

Meulemann, H. 2001. "Life Satisfaction from Late Adolescence to Mid-Life." *Journal of Happiness Studies* 2 (4): 445–65.

Meyers, S., and S. Landsberger. 2002. "Direct and Indirect Pathways Between Adult Attachment Style and Marital Satisfaction." *Personal Relationships* 9 (2): 159–72.

Michalos, A., and B. Zumbo. 1999. "Public Services and the Quality of Life." *Social Indicators Research* 48 (2): 125–56.

Morman, M., and K. Floyd. 2002. "A 'Changing Culture of Fatherhood': Effects on Affectionate Communication, Closeness, and Satisfaction in Men's Relationships with Their Fathers and Their Sons." *Western Journal of Communication* 66 (4): 395–411.

Mowrer, R., and D. McCarver. 2002. "A Preliminary Investigation of Multicultural Perspective and Life Satisfaction." *Psychological Reports* 90 (1): 251–56.

Mueller, D., and K. Kim. 2004. "The Tenacious Goal Pursuit and Flexible Goal Adjustment Scales: Examination of Their Validity." *Educational and Psychological Measurement* 64 (1): 120–42.

Nair, E. 2000. "Health and Aging." *Journal of Adult Development* 7 (2): 121–26.

Olsson, H., H. Backe, S. Soerensen, and M. Kock. 2002. "The Essence of Humor and Its Effects and Functions: A Qualitative Study." *Journal of Nursing Management* 10 (1): 21–26.

Othaganont, P., C. Sinthuvorakan, and P. Jensupakarn. 2002. "Daily Living Practice of the Life-Satisfied Thai Elderly." *Journal of Transcultural Nursing* 13 (1): 24–29.

Palmore, E., and V. Kivett. 1977. "Change in Life Satisfaction: A Longitudinal Study of Persons Aged 46–70." *Journal of Gerontology* 32 (3): 311–16.

Peterson, C. 1999. "Grandfathers' and Grandmothers' Satisfaction with the Grandparenting Role: Seeking New Answers to Old Questions." *International Journal of Aging and Human Development* 49 (1): 61–78.

Pinkleton, B., and E. Austin. 2002. "Exploring Relationships Among Media Use Frequency, Perceived Media Importance, and Media Satisfaction in Political Disaffection and Efficacy." *Mass Communication and Society* 5 (2): 141–63.

Prezza, M., M. Amici, T. Roberti, and G. Tedeschi. 2001. "Sense of Community Referred to the Whole Town: Its Relations with Neighboring, Loneliness, Life Satisfaction, and Area of Residence." *Journal of Community Psychology* 29 (1): 29–52.

Reboussin, B., W. J. Rejeski, K. Martin, and K. Callahan. 2000. "Correlates of Satisfaction with Body Function and Body Appearance in Middle- and Older-Aged Adults." *Psychology and Health* 15 (2): 239–54.

Reis-Bergan, M., F. Gibbons, M. Gerrard, and J. Ybema. 2000. "The Impact of Reminiscence on Socially Active Elderly Women's Reactions to Social Comparisons." *Basic and Applied Social Psychology* 22 (3): 225–36.

Reitzes, D., and E. Mutran. 2002. "Self-Concept as the Organization of Roles: Importance, Centrality, and Balance." *Sociological Quarterly* 43 (4): 647–67.

Richardson, R., and A. Sistler. 1999. "The Well-Being of Elderly Black Caregivers and Noncaregivers." *Journal of Gerontological Social Work* 31 (1–2): 109–17.

Richburg, M. 1998. "The Relationship Between Dyadic Adjustment and the Structure, Satisfaction, and Intimacy of Married Men's Same-Sex Friendships." Ph.D. dissertation, University of Denver.

Riggs, A., and B. Turner. 2000. "Pie-Eyed Optimists: Baby-Boomers, the Optimistic Generation?" *Social Indicators Research* 52 (1): 73–93.

Robinson-Rowe, M. 2002. "Meaning and Satisfaction in the Lives of Midlife, Never-Married Heterosexual Women." Ph.D. dissertation, Alliant International University.

Rosen-Grandon, J., J. Myers, and J. Hattie. 2004. "The Relationship Between Marital Characteristics, Marital Interaction Processes, and Marital Satisfaction." *Journal of Counseling and Development* 82 (1): 58–68.

Ryan, L., and S. Dziurawiec. 2001. "Materialism and Its Relationship to Life Satisfaction." *Social Indicators Research* 55 (2): 185–97.

Sarkisian, C., and R. Hays, S. Berry, and C. Mangione. 2001. "Expectations Regarding Aging Among Older Adults and Physicians Who Care for Older Adults." *Medical Care* 39 (9): 1025–36.

Scannell, E., F. Allen, and J. Burton. 2002. "Meaning in Life and Positive and Negative Well-Being." *North American Journal of Psychology* 4 (1): 93–112.

Schiffman, L., E. Sherman, and M. Long. 2003. "Toward a Better Understanding of the Interplay of Personal Values and the Internet." *Psychology and Marketing* 20 (2): 169–86.

Shackelford, T., and D. Buss. 2000. "Marital Satisfaction and Spousal Cost-Infliction." *Personality and Individual Differences* 28 (5): 917–28.

Simons, C. 2002. "Proactive Coping, Perceived Self-Efficacy, and Locus of Control as Predictors of Life Satisfaction in Young, Middle-Aged, and Older Adults." Ph.D. dissertation, Georgia State University.

Stacey, C., A. Kozma, and M. Stones. 1985. "Simple Cognitive and Behavioral Changes Resulting from Improved Physical Fitness in Persons over 50 Years of Age." *Canadian Journal on Aging* 4 (2): 67–74.

Thompson, L., M. Aidinejad, and J. Ponte. 2001. "Aging and the Effects of Facial and Prosodic Cues on Emotional Intensity Ratings and Memory Reconstructions." *Journal of Nonverbal Behavior* 25 (2): 101–25.

Timmerman, G., and G. Acton. 2001. "The Relationship Between Basic Need Satisfaction and Emotional Eating." *Issues in Mental Health Nursing* 22 (7): 691–701.

Van Handel Eagles, J. 1999. " An Inquiry into the Incidence and Nature of Mentoring Relationships in Women over the Age of Sixty." Ph.D. dissertation, Walden University.

Van Willigen, M. 2000. "Differential Benefits of Volunteering Across the Life Course." *Journals of Gerontology: Psychological Sciences and Social Sciences* 55 (5): 308–18.

Waldrop, D., and J. Weber. 2001. "From Grandparent to Caregiver: The Stress and Satisfaction of Raising Grandchildren." *Families in Society* 82 (5): 461–72.

Wallace, K., T. Bisconti, and C. Bergeman. 2001. "The Mediational Effect of Hardiness on Social Support and Optimal Outcomes in Later Life." *Basic and Applied Social Psychology* 23 (4): 267–79.

Warr, P., V. Butcher, and I. Robertson. 2004. "Activity and Psychological Well-Being in Older People." *Aging and Mental Health* 8 (2): 172–83.

Weaver, C. 2003. "Happiness of Mexican Americans." *Hispanic Journal of Behavioral Sciences* 25 (3): 275–94.

Weigel, D., and D. Ballard-Reisch. 1999. "All Marriages Are Not Maintained Equally: Marital Type, Marital Quality, and the Use of Maintenance Behaviors." *Personal Relationships* 6 (3): 291–303.

Weigel, D., K. Bennett, and S. Ballard-Reisch. 2003. "Family Influences on Commitment: Examining the Family of Origin Correlates of Relationship Commitment Attitudes." *Personal Relationships* 10 (4): 453–74.

Wells, Y., and H. Kendig. 1999. "Psychological Resources and Successful Retirement." *Australian Psychologist* 34 (2): 111–15.

Westerhof, G., F. Dittmann-Kohli, and T. Thissen. 2001. "Beyond Life Satisfaction: Lay Conceptions of Well-Being Among Middle-Aged and Elderly Adults." *Social Indicators Research* 56 (2): 179–203.

Winslow, L., 2001. "The Relationship of Gambling on Depression, Perceived Social Support, and Life Satisfaction in an Elderly Sample." Ph.D. dissertation, Hofstra University.

Yamada, N. 2000. "The Relationship Between Leisure Activities, Psycho-Social Development and Life Satisfaction in Late Adulthood." *Japanese Journal of Developmental Psychology* 11 (1): 34–44.

Zhou, J., and J. George. 2001. "When Job Dissatisfaction Leads to Creativity: Encouraging the Expression of Voice." *Academy of Management Journal* 44 (4): 682–96.